I0471339

In Sickness and In Health

A Husbands Story of Surviving Breast Cancer

Michael Streicker

Copyright © 2013 Michael Streicker

All rights reserved.

ISBN:1489510362
ISBN-13: 978-1489510365

DEDICATION

This book is dedicated to my beautiful wife Jen.

Because you are so amazing that there should be a new word for you.

Jamazing.

Jamazing is when you do something so awesome, so tough, so powerful, that it can only be done by you.

You are Jamazing.

I love you.

CHAPTERS

ACKNOWLEDGMENTS

I would like to thank my lovely wife Jennifer for supporting this project even though revisiting certain topics was stressful for her. And to all the people that have helped us through it for all of these years, thank you.

1 INTRODUCTION

My wife was diagnosed with stage 1 breast cancer. We will talk as we go along about how and when we found it and what we have been through since she was diagnosed. I decided to write this book, after sitting back and thinking about what we had been through and how much it, well, basically….sucked. Most of the books we had read were of little help. They mostly focused on how breast cancer would make her or both of us better people or that she was supposed to get in touch with her inner womanhoodness, or other things that few people under 50 years old, believe in. We realized early on that there were no support groups for couples, let alone for young couples trying to make it through this. We were really surprised by that. Then there were these things called husbands which really nobody talked about in the world of breast cancer. I know that sounds bitter or angry but it is not meant to do so. It is just an honest assessment of the state of things when my wife was diagnosed with breast cancer and it remains the same many years later. We wholly support the momentum behind the breast cancer support groups, charities, and research that is being done today and believe that the publicity that it gets is wonderful. But it leaves out large groups of people like husbands and it does not talk about or focus on actually living day to day through the whole ordeal. Most of the books, groups, etc. focus on your "spirit" and "woman power". Great concepts for some people but I would be willing to bet that most folks are focused on getting up tomorrow and making it through the day rather than planning their next hike in the mountains to commune with mother earth. We did eventually find a group that really has helped her find functional tools that help her, and me, on a day to day basis. But it took years to find that and they are only at a few hospitals in the whole country. And for something that affects a large number of women, it by definition affects a large number of men as well. For other things such as drug and alcohol abuse, there are support groups for the families. For breast cancer? Not much. As focused as we should be on saving the lives of the women diagnosed, something needs to be done for those of us who hold their heads while they puke and get them pain meds at 4 am.

More than anything else, that last part is
why I am writing this. Because for a
disease that affects so many women, it
affects a lot of men as well. This is in no
way meant to take away or diminish the
physical or mental suffering the women
under treatment for breast cancer endure. I
would have then and still would do
anything for Jen not to have gone through
that situation. If I could have taken her
place on the table or the other side of the
needle, I would not have hesitated to do so.
But my point is that there is so much
support and attention already given to that
group (the patient), that I felt there should
be a little bit of time spent on what the
couple and the husband specifically goes
through when breast cancer invades your
marriage.

A lot of this book covers things that I
have found to be helpful and that
hopefully you will as well. Things that
helped her eat better, maybe cry a little
less, or just be more comfortable when the
pain hit. By helping her, it helps us. The
hardest thing in all of this has been
watching her suffering in pain, and not
being able in some cases to do anything

about it. Anytime I could alleviate it by any means necessary, I was willing to do so. I thoroughly believe that if you are reading this book, you feel that way about your wife as well.

This is not self-help book. It is not a cathartic book to help me or the two of us feel better about the things we have been through. It sucked then, looking back it still sucks, and I don't really recommend that anyone try it for fun or for a reality TV series. More than anything else, I wrote this so that other husbands know that they are not alone in the feelings they may be having, decisions they have to make, or the situations that they are unsure of how to handle. So that maybe the couples who do not have the communication that my lovely wife and I have in our marriage, can use this book to help them talk about issues they have avoided talking about. There are a lot of issues that have to be dealt with in the process that nobody wants to talk about openly like dealing with family, fertility, the sudden lack of sex life, potential physical and emotional scars, and how to keep your marriage together through breast cancer.

As you read through the book, the chapters were written by me, with the editing and input of my wife. Originally, we were going to write the book together. We were going to pick topics and write both sides of it. I started my part and when she tried to do the same, it was just too emotional for her to do so. It hasn't been easy for me either but I felt strongly that it needed to be done so I powered through. So it has ended up being pretty much my side of things. But she has helped me greatly by reminding me of a few things to add, pointing out things that she did not want the public to visualize about her or us, and by listening to my thoughts and feelings along the way.

I really felt that part was important because, just as many men do not like to talk about their feelings, we do not always really hear what our wives are saying

either. I believe this to be a rare
phenomena but Jen tells me otherwise.
The chronology is also somewhat helter-
skelter. Some chapters go in
chronological order and some follow a
single subject matter through the whole
process. Some of this is just our story and
I hope that you never have to deal with
anything like it and other parts hopefully
are useful to anyone willing to read it.

I am sure that something in this book will
offend you or make you say "I would
never think/feel/say that!", but I am going
to be as open and honest as my wife
would let me be. It is not meant to offend
people and I am not here to put down or
belittle anyone else's situation or opinion.
But I am here to defend my right to an
opinion as someone who has been through
it and to stimulate others into expressing
their feelings and opinions when
especially husbands may not always be
encouraged to do so. You have to be a
part of the process, help make decisions,
and be a part of the team. Others are there

to help and you will need them. But it has
to be you in her corner at the end of every
round. That means there could be strong
language, maybe some sexual content,
and definitely a lot of adult situations. As
we say in our house "Man Up" and read.

2 WHAT THE HELL IS THAT?

We had just come home from New Jersey
and our yearly New Year's gathering with
friends the weekend before. The house
was a mess after Christmas and there were
decorations and presents all over the
place. We were putting all of this away
and Jen was handing things to me to put
in the attic when she leaned a box onto
her chest to get better hand hold to hand it
up to me. Ouch! That did not feel right.
Jen felt pain in her left breast and when
we finished putting things away, she
stopped to examine the area. She found a
little swollen lump. I checked it out as
well since I generally do not turn down
the actual invitation to touch my wife and
confirmed that it was a little swollen
lump. We talked about it, figured it was
nothing but we should get it checked out.

Since both of us are scientists and work in
biomedical and cancer research, we
realized that there are all sorts of bumps
in your body that are no big deal. But you

see, we had been trying for about 6 months to get pregnant and Jen had recently started taking some low level fertility drugs to help out in the process. They told us to watch for any weird things happening in her body so we figured that was what it was. No biggie, but let's tell somebody anyway.

Jen went in to see her OBGYN and he told her it was probably a cyst but to go see a surgeon about it to be sure. That was on Monday. On Wednesday, we went to see the surgeon and he attempted to do a fine needle biopsy in the office. That did not do much. He was not able to get any fluid out which meant that a cyst was less likely and Jen thought it was horribly painful when they stuck the little needle into her breast. Although, looking back on it at how much "pain" that Jen was in for the procedure, it seems very trivial now.

The surgeon said we could keep an eye on it or go ahead and schedule a lumpectomy to see what it was. We both felt that the best way to go was to take it out and went forward with that plan.

So here is the part where I give a little mini-lecture/tirade (don't worry, you will get used to them) about not "keeping an eye on it". Luckily, Jen's surgeon likes to err on the side of caution and agreed with our idea of just yanking the lump out. However, this is where things can go to hell in a hand basket. A lot of people that we talked to that had advanced breast cancer or positive lymph nodes, etc., were the ones that opted to wait and see what happened in the same situation we were in. They were busy or the holidays were coming up, they couldn't take time off of work, etc. Guess what…..you should not wait and see….ever. I don't care who's coming to dinner on Saturday night or if Susie is the Pumpkin in the school play. Stop whatever you are doing and have it taken out and checked. If it is nothing….great…..you win. If it is cancer….YOU GOT IT OUT OF YOUR BODY! Yeah, you will need more treatment and testing but like I learned as a kid…"Knowing is half the battle". And the earlier you get it diagnosed, the better your chances are and the less ugly it will hopefully be in the long run. There have been so many people that have told us that their doctors told them not to bother taking it out and really leaned on them to just watch it for a few weeks or months. Some had to go see another doctor for a 2nd opinion before they found one to have it removed. And many of those were positive for cancer. Yes, the percentages may be low but if you are one of those 3%, no good came out of watching it. Early detection does save lives. So does taking control of your own healthcare.

Jen had the lumpectomy the following week and we waited for the results. All of the people so far had told us that there was very little chance that it would be cancerous. This was statistically true, doctors yank lumps, bumps, and cysts out of people all day everyday and it is generally no big deal. Until it comes back as cancer for you or someone you love. My wife was young, only 29, and with no family history.

The first surgery was at a nearby hospital that was luckily about 2 miles from our house. A brand new and very nice facility where she ended up having most of her surgeries. We went in that morning nervous but truly expecting that it was just a cyst or something and not a big deal. This was before we had IPod's so I packed up my bag with a book to read, a CD player, and a stack of CD's to listen to as I waited. One of the big issues that day was whether we needed to have a dozen people at the hospital. I really did not want or need anyone to sit with me and we just really wanted to get it out and go home quietly that day. Of that whole year, that day is more of a blur than any other because it was when we still thought Jen was cancer free and it was going to be a one and done situation. They called her in and she had a quick surgery and I took her home. She struggles with anesthesia so she was crying as she came out and demanding her Chapstick but other than that, it was a pretty uneventful day. At this point, we had not really told many

people about the surgery. Just my
parents, her mother, and her brothers and
one or two friends. We did not think it
was going to amount to anything so we
did not make it a big deal. Wishful
thinking on our part.

Here is one place you need to sort of start
deciding who you tell things to because
the rumors will start and then you have to
deal with people being offended that they
did not know earlier. I am not saying to
call an early press conference but just
something to keep in mind. Each of you
has a different dynamic in your family
and circle of friends. You will have to
make that decision for yourselves.

3 MIKE FINDS OUT

We were in the middle of an ice storm which living in the southern part of the USA will shut things down faster than a health code violation. But, being a Northerner and driver of a Jeep, I was at work and was hosting a week long client visit that could not be rescheduled. The doctors' appointment that we had scheduled to find out the results had been changed due to the storm, but our surgeon was kind enough to agree to call us as soon as he was able to get the pathology report faxed to his home. He got it, read it, and called Jen at home.

I got paged out of the meeting by Jen's phone call. She told me that the doctor had called and then she started to cry. When Jen said "I have cancer" my heart sank. Not the words I expected to hear. For Christ's sake, we were 29 years old and all around pretty healthy people. Well, shit. I was standing in a room with several other people and I had to go right back into a meeting and put on a happy business face for the staff and client. All I wanted to do was curl up in a ball and cry. I was able, as I have had too much practice doing in my life, to ball it up and tuck it under the rug until I was able to get through the day.

I got everything done and got into my Jeep and made it about halfway home before pulling off into a shopping mall parking lot and balling my eyes out. It just hit me and I could not breathe. What the fuck had happened here? My wife, the one thing in this world that I love beyond words and that I could truly not live without had a deadly disease. This was some bullshit. I was so scared and so mad at the same time. I had lost too much and too damn many people in my life for this to happen. I had lost a niece, and a brother, a close friend from college, and I had always had a reoccurring nightmare since childhood that I would lose my wife young. I was in shambles for about 15 minutes.

I also realized that I could not go home in

that kind of shape or Jen would not be able to handle it. I knew that she needed me to be the strong one at the moment so I got myself together and finished the drive home.

By the time I got there, Jen's brothers were both there. They had driven down from Washington DC when they got the call from Jen. I dearly love my brother-in-laws, nobody…flat out nobody could ask for better. They were understanding about it and when I got there, they left the room to give Jen and me some time to cry and talk since we had not seen each other since finding out. At that point we had no plan or ability to even formulate one. We just sat in our bed with our dogs and cried and talked about what a bad deal we had just gotten. By the end of the day, more family had shown up at the house from DC and Jen's best friend had come in from the coast.

That night, we basically just tried to

accept what had happened and start to come up with a plan. My wife and I are very "plan" oriented people. Plus it was something to focus on besides crying. We started thinking about what we knew about breast cancer and how we wanted to start the process of finding doctors and researching treatment options.

4 FOLLOW THE YELLOW BRICK ROAD

Two days later we embarked on a series of doctors' appointments that seemed never ending. We agreed early on to see three of each type of specialist before choosing one to go forward with. This gave us a chance to compare the individual doctors, their staff and facilities, and get some very varied opinions on treatment. We happen to live in an area of the country that is dripping in hospitals and rank with the best in the world so we had plenty of options. The one exception that we made was in the surgeon that we choose.

By chance, the surgeon that we had been referred to by Jen's Obstetrician/Gynecologist was great. We were in such a hurry to get the first surgery done that we did not bother to get a second opinion as we were both fairly knowledgeable on the subject and agreed with him on the surgery. After the first surgery, the combination of intelligence, skill, bedside manner, and results (superficial scarring) that he showed us made it easy to not look elsewhere. I have dealt with many doctors and surgeons in my life and he is by far, the best I have ever met. Very seldom in this world do you find people that you instantly trust and treat you with respect and caring from the first time you meet them. He is one of those people and we are incredibly thankful that we were lucky enough to have him as our surgeon. Since I do not want to mention specific names and places in the book, he will be known in these pages as Dr. Surgery.

We next had to pick an oncologist. The first one that we met with was very eye opening. We had just found out about this issue two days prior and were still in shock and disbelief on many levels. When we walked into the office and saw the patients waiting to go in for chemotherapy, it was incredibly difficult to even stay there for our appointment. There was nothing wrong with anything we saw there; it was all very newly furbished and high tech. But we were still somewhat in denial of the situation. We were in no way ready for hair falling out as patients sat there, or people barely able to get out of the chairs by themselves. Jen was crushed by what she saw. One of the hardest things to do when you are in the throes of the situation is to realize that (hopefully) you might not be as bad off as the person you are looking at. That maybe you will get a different treatment. The doctor was very nice but we knew there was no chance of us choosing him because of the eye-popping and acute reality that had just set in for both of us. There was just no way to wash away that initial memory and smack in the face so we just could not go back there.

The next oncologist that we saw was also very nice. He was in an established practice and had a very good reputation. He was in the running, except for his view on fertility after chemotherapy. He felt that it was not something that we should even consider and did not really want to talk about it. He basically told us that

having children was really never going to
happen for us and that was a huge blow
for Jen. His position was that you should
just try to get through the breast cancer
and that if you did so, just be happy to be
alive and don't worry about trying to have
kids. Considering the fact that until a few
days ago we were actively trying to do
just that very thing, it was not what we
needed to hear at that time.

The third oncologist that we saw was a
woman at a major university hospital.
This was a massive clinic that was world
renowned for its care and research. Jen
and I both work in the cancer research
field and this doctor was referred to us
from several sources for being a leader in
the research field and being on the front
line of the breast cancer fight. We could
tell from the start that she definitely knew
her stuff. She was open to the idea of
having kids one day and said that she
would work with us on that when the time
came. At the same time, she annoyed me
because she kept using the phrase "the
research shows…." But I would ask her
for the paper or reference and she did not

particularly like me questioning her about it. Once we saw her, Jen instantly decided that she was the one that she wanted to go with for an oncologist. I had some reservations about it because we had to wait a very long time to get in that day and it was by far the longest drive from the house but Jen was adamant about wanting this doctor so that is who we went with.

The next specialist that we went to see was the plastic surgeon. We first saw a surgeon that specialized in cancer and burn patients. Again, he was nice enough but the patients in the office were in really bad shape and this was difficult to handle at that point. He had a book of pictures to show us of patients that had various different breast cancer reconstruction procedures done. For those of you that are not aware, there are several different types of reconstruction options available to most women. We will discuss this more in another chapter. We were not particularly pleased with the results he showed us as his examples. Not that he was a bad surgeon or that the pictures were drastically different from others that we saw but again, for the first time seeing the results, it was extremely difficult. Part of the problem was that the pictures were all from probably two to six weeks post surgery. If any doctors are out there reading this, it would really help people if you could do six month to two years post surgery follow up pictures. I realize that it might be hard to get people to come back at that point but just a couple of pictures would be nice to see the light at the end of the tunnel. He also wanted to do what is called a Tram-Flap procedure that neither of us was all that interested in. He was insistent about that procedure being performed in Jen's case because that was the "new" thing in breast reconstruction at that point. So that sort of took him out of the running.

The next plastic surgeon (Dr. Plastics) that we saw was not a cancer specialist but did reconstructions as well as general boob jobs. A friend of ours had a mole removed by him and just dropped his name to us. It was literally right down the street so we figured we would check him out. His office was like something out of a movie. We went in and all of the other patients were strippers, rich housewives who wanted to look like strippers or 15 year old girls who wanted to be strippers. It could not have been more drastically different that the last office we saw. There was leather furniture with a fireplace in the waiting room. We went back to see him and he was exactly the right fit for us. He was very honest, funny, and willing to work with us on the whole plan. He looked at Jen's breasts and asked her what cup size she was and what cup size she would like to be. He told us that if we wanted to "upgrade" it would be very easy to do. One of the best quotes of the year for us was when he looked at Jen and said "Now Jen, you're a big girl, you can handle bigger breasts." That sealed the deal for us. Not that she wanted to Super Size necessarily but he was just our type of person.

The third plastic surgeon that we saw was back at the major university hospital. We were pretty positive that we wanted to use Dr. Plastics but the oncologist we chose felt that nobody was better than the people at the university and she insisted that we see a surgeon and plastic surgeon from that staff. We saw both. The problem that we had there was a long wait time to get in to see each of them and the single agenda (Tram-Flap) that they wanted to perform. It was a slightly different version of it than the first plastic surgeon that we had seen but still they did not want to consider implants which we felt was the best option to us.

The doctors from the university hospital were nice but we felt that we wanted very much to stay with Dr. Surgery and to choose Dr. Plastics. The really good thing about the surgeons that we choose was that they worked at the hospital that was 1 mile from our house. The others were a 30 minute drive away.

Time for another mini-lecture. In no way,

shape, or form, are we suggesting any given treatment or surgical option over another for anyone else's case but our situation. We realize that each case is different and each couple is different. What we chose may seem silly to someone else and vice versa. What I will adamantly demand of each of you is that you really think about the options you are given and understand what they mean for you. Two surgeons may call a procedure the same thing but mean something slightly different. Those small differences could mean a lot to you in the long run. We saw three plastic surgeons that gave us pretty drastically different viewpoints and surgical plans. I can't say that would be the case for everybody but if you do not like what you hear, ask somebody else. Maybe they will give you another option you like better. Maybe they will tell you the exact same thing as the first doctor. But at least you will know. Doctors and surgeons are highly educated and trained people but that does not mean that you should have blind faith in everything that they tell you. Do your research and ask questions. You will be

with these people a lot in the coming
years so you should feel comfortable
asking them things and they should be
respectful in their answers. A lot of "just
trust me" statements from them should
really make you think about seeing
someone else. I realize that we were a
little ahead of the game because we are
both in the sciences and do research so we
understood a lot of the terminology and
processes. But even if you do not have a
science background, you can and should
learn the terminology of cancer and take
notes so that you can investigate things
later. Just remember that not everything
on the internet is true.

One of the best decisions that we made in
the whole process was that we were going
to make each decision together, go to
every possible appointment together, and
not to discuss anything with others that
we had not first discussed with each other.
This was very important because we were
able to bounce things off of each other
and discuss things and make decisions, as
we normally do, together. There were
people around us that wanted to go to

appointments and have a say or vote in what we decided to do. They wanted to enforce their agenda on the process but we made it clear that we were the starters on the team and there was no bench. It meant that we hurt some people's feelings from time to time during that period but we were the ones who had to deal most acutely with the consequences of our decisions so we felt that we needed to make them together and not as a part of any larger committees.

5 TELLING FAMILY AND FRIENDS

One of the things that we had originally decided when we were first diagnosed and started the process of getting this lump checked out was that we were not telling much to anybody. We did not think it was going to be cancer and therefore did not want to get people scared or worried. It was not until we had a positive cancer diagnosis that we told anybody other than immediate family. In truth, we had a long discussion about not telling them either but we decided it would cause too much trouble down the line regardless of the outcome.

When you have something like this happen, everybody wants to be involved and help somehow. Some people send flowers and cards. This is very nice but when it starts to look like a funeral home, it is out of hand. Jen kept every card that she got sent in a couple of baskets in our living room. Very large baskets. She, and I say she because 98% were addressed to her, got over 300 cards over the course of the year. We also got care packages that included anything from puzzles and crosswords to gift cards to rent movies and go to dinner. We received enough movie rental gift cards that we did not pay for a movie for over 9 months. And we rent a lot of movies. We also received hundreds of dollars in gift cards to various restaurants. Most of our family and friends are spread coast to coast over the whole country so many of these came from people unfamiliar with the area were we lived. So they went to the internet and searched for restaurants in our town. It turns out that geographically, Applebee's was the closest restaurant to us. So we got a LOT of Applebee's gift cards. Up to that point, we had honestly never eaten there. It is kind of tucked behind another store and we did not truly know it was there. We have since become well-acquainted. The generosity that was shown by people during that year was amazing. There were people that sent a card every week, and people who sent flowers or gift cards on a regular basis. It was very overwhelming to think about

how many people in the world cared
about us specifically.

One of the things that was very hard to do
for us was to call people and keep them
updated. It was hard to make 8 phone
calls and relay the exact same information
after each appointment or treatment.
Much less field the calls of the next 25
people in line to find out what was
happening. At the same time, one of the
big problems that we had early on was
inaccurate information being spread that
made things out to be much worse than it
actually was. It's like the telephone game
you play as a kid where you sit in a circle
and whisper a story to the person next to
you and by the time it comes back around,
it is pretty much a different story. Maybe
people were just hard to understand
because they were crying and upset or
maybe people just embellished here and
there but we got some frantic calls from
those who had heard that Jen was all but
dead. We put the word out to please stop
calling us because it was just too draining
but we also wanted to make sure that
people heard the right information without

deputizing anyone else to speak for us.
We decided to make an e-mail list of all
of the people that we felt should be aware
of the situation. This list included family
and friends of ours and also other people
we were asked to add by our family and
friends. I sent out updates as we
progressed through treatments and
surgeries. Sometimes I sent them out to
just let people know we were chugging
along but nothing had changed. This
helped us greatly by reducing the amount
of time that we had to spend on the phone
and it also helped to make sure that
everybody got the real information. With
the social networking websites like
Facebook and others, you can disseminate
information quickly to lots of people if
you set it up right. I know it sounds
somewhat impersonal but I promise that
after you spend a couple of days doing it
the old fashion way, it will wear you out.

So one of the first things that happens
when you find out that your wife has
breast cancer is that everybody you are

related to, close friends, and people that
you once bought peaches from on the side
of the road, want to help you somehow.
And they want to be there. At your house.
"Helping". My wife and I are not really
what you would call a needy couple. My
wife would generally qualify as needy but
she married me to take care of her and I
tend to be an enabler so it works out most
of the time. We love our families and
friends and spend a lot of time with them
normally. But we take very good care of
ourselves and have a certain way that we
live our life and run our house. We work
a lot and I play rugby more or less all year
which means that we are rarely home at
the same time for more than a few hours
so we try to do most things around the
house together. We do our grocery
shopping together on Friday nights and
then we put them away and go out to the
movies. We put laundry away together.
We clean the house together while we
crank music through the stereo. And a lot
of the time, we lie on the couch with our
dogs and watch TV. That all goes to shit
when you basically open a bed and
breakfast for breast cancer. We had more
"help" than we really knew what to do

with. We understood that this was all
meant to be good and to be helpful but it
was, in its own way, disruptive as well.
When you are going through a lot of
stress, it is nice to have a safe place where
things are normal. It is nice to be able to
come back and talk to each other and
make decisions before people start in with
the questions and want a play by play of
everything that was said and done. We
did not always have that option. We often
would go out to lunch or dinner after an
appointment because we needed to talk
before we went home and held a press
conference.

Things got rearranged in our kitchen and
put places making it difficult to find
things like a spatula. We did not cook
very often at that point as we both either
worked late or had other things going on,
so our refrigerator was not well stocked
with actual food. Any condiment that you
ever wanted plus cookie mix and cheese
but not a lot of stuff to cook dinner. This
was remedied when people went shopping

and bought a fridge full of food that was either things we do not eat or "all-natural organic" things that smelled like feet. But they were convinced that Jen got cancer from our eating habits. Another visitor did not like our frying pans so they went out and bought us new ones and took our olds ones away. Great that we got new frying pans but again, not as helpful in practice as it probably was conceived to be in theory. We understood that people wanted to help and to do what they could to make our lives a little easier. We appreciated all of it, but it was also hard to accept or maybe just different than what we would have done sometimes.

We decided that we were instituting a "no means no" policy when it came to people coming over or visiting us. We had problems with telling people no and then having them show up anyway. We did our best to put a stop to that and it worked well with a few exceptions. We did have a lot of visitors during the year and we enjoyed it very much for the most part. Many of the people who came would have come normally but did so more often than normal. So we got to see our friends and family more than we normally do which is mostly a good thing.

We also had a rule that our safe house was our bedroom. Nobody went in there to clean, put clothes away, or anything else, unless we asked them to do so. This was important because we needed to have someplace to keep "normal". Some people have a habit of taking over no matter the situation and ignoring rules that are not theirs. They would repeatedly go into our bedroom and open the blinds "to let the healing light in". This pissed me off incredibly and did not set well with Jen either. We like our bedroom dark. It is a little cave that our family (us and the dogs) can sleep and cuddle (dogs too). So we made and enforced the rule. It took us a little while but we eventually gained control of our own home.

Like I said, this is a difficult balance to keep. You do not want to offend the

people there to help you and may really
need help from at some point. But you
also need to keep things the way you and
your wife need them to be in order to cope
with everything else you have going on. I
would really suggest that you try to be
proactive about what things you and your
wife would find "helpful" and then clearly
communicate your needs and wants.

It was equally difficult when Jen had
surgeries or treatments and various people
wanted to come and be there. This was
particularly hard for us because we did
not want to offend people, for example
her mom and brothers and my parents,
that all offered and wanted to be there
while she was in surgery to make sure she
was O.K. and also to keep me company
all day at the hospital. Uh yeah….so let
me put it this way. Most of you reading
this book, probably 99.99% don't know
me from Adam. The one's who do know
me, know this: the last place you want to
be is next to Mike when he is pissed off
and worried about Jen. I give our family
props for caring and wanting to be there
but I really more than anything wanted to

be left alone. I don't even sit in the waiting room with strangers. I just don't like people that much. I sit in a corner where I can listen to music and read. And easily find a smoking area. Lots of smoking that year (I have since quit, I heard it was bad for you). Anyway, people came and went and I was not much fun to be around and mostly avoided them at the hospital. I am telling you this because you need to remember that you have the right to do what you need to do to handle the situation. If you like having a ton of people there...do it. Believe me, there was someone having a mole removed that had 10 people in the waiting room. But if you need to have your space, just say so. Try to be nice and explain how you feel (I did try), but do what you have to do to get through the day. You have to realize that they are going through this as well and balance that into your decisions but you also have to take care of you.

One of the biggest things you learn when

you go through this is who your friends really are and what friendship means to you and them. We are incredibly lucky to have some very good friends. We have always known that but it was reinforced that year and in the years to follow.

One of our close friends lost his father to a heart attack during the same time Jen was going through one of her surgeries, but he stilled called to check on her. It was actually very hard for us because we would normally have dropped what we were doing and driven up to be with him for the funeral. It was difficult for me not to be there for one of my closest friends but he threatened to shoot me if I left Jen at home to come to the funeral. And he owns a lot of guns.

A big mistake that we made was that we did not tell a couple that are very close friends of ours but were due with their first baby the week after Jen's first surgery. They called to tell us the news of their daughters' birth the day we got Jen's diagnosis. We held off telling them

because we did not want to take away
from their happiness.
Ummmm....yeah.....I did not know that
they knew some of the words they called
us when we finally told them and they
discovered we had held out on them.

We did not discover this until later but
there is a website called Caring Bridge
that works more or less like a blog. You
can post updates to it and people can read
them and also post comments and
encouragement. It is a great way to get
information out to a semi-controlled
group.

We can't thank our friends and family
enough for all of the things that they did
to help us get through that year and the
years and trials that have followed. Yes,
there were some things I would not do if I
were on the other side but we could not
have made it without help. We are
incredibly lucky to have the kind of
family that we do and the friends that we

have. When things start to fall apart, it is good when you know who you can really count on. We know that we have no shortage of people to turn to.

It is not particularly easy for me to accept help or to let others do things for me or Jen. I just like to be self reliant which did not always make things easy when you have others trying very hard to help. In particular, Jen's mother and I did not see eye to eye during parts of the process. When two people love someone as much as a mother/husband love a daughter/wife, it can be very hard to not get in each other's way. She and I definitely had our moments during these years, but we made it through and I think gained something in our relationship because of it. I think few mothers love their children as much as she does and even fewer offer more help to their children in life. She dropped whatever she had going on to come down whenever we asked, always offered even when we said we had it covered, and tried to respect our needs as well as her own.

By the same token, I probably offended
my own parents by asking them not to
come to the hospital for surgeries. But I
found it very hard to be around others
when I really only wanted to be around
my wife. I was very single minded and
thought only of her and us throughout
most of the process. I was not too terribly
concerned for the needs of others in the
process and looking back, I could have
done some things differently to help
others deal with the stress as well.

I know that for most of us, the first
reaction is to protect and shelter our
wives. I am all for that. But what was the
hardest for me was to let go enough that
other people who felt the need to protect
and shelter her could do so. I am sure I
did not do a particularly good job of
letting other's (Jen's brothers, her mother,
my parents, and others) have their turn in
protecting and sheltering her during that
first year. If so, I do apologize and I hope
that as readers, you can keep this in mind
when you are going through this for

yourselves. It may sound bad but it may be best for everybody if you went fishing and let someone else make her lunch. It gives you a break from caring for her which while you will say you don't want or need it, you probably do. And it lets someone else help when they so desperately want to do so.

I feel that our dogs also really deserve some very special recognition for the role they have played in this. O.K., yes they are dogs and do not (that I have seen them) read but still, we could not have made it through without them.

One of the things that really upsets Jen and I is when people have pets that are treated like second class citizens in the house. Seriously…get fish if that is what you want in a pet. Our dogs are family. They are our son and daughter and always will be.

They picked up quickly that something was wrong with their mom and acted accordingly. They were so gentle and loving to her that it was astounding. Anyone who says they can't feel emotion like that or should not be allowed near a sick person is an idiot. They kept watch over Jen and cared for her almost as much as I did those years. When she was sick on the floor of the bathroom, they would curl up against her to comfort her. I saw them get up when she would be shivering and cold and go lay against her before I could even get up to get a blanket.

We used to have my dog and her dog but mine abandoned me that year to watch over Jen. They were with her constantly. When I would come home, they would meet me at the door and then lead me directly to wherever she was at the time to check on her. Anytime she cried, which was a lot that year, they would go and sit with her and let her cry into their fur if I was not there. Again, you may think it strange but I am as thankful for them and what they did for us that year as I am anybody else. I just feel that the role that

animals can play in our lives is a great one
and I would discourage you from keeping
your dog out of the process because of
fear of germs or some such nonsense.

Our happy place is definitely on the
couch or in bed with our dogs and we use
it a lot.

6 WOULD YOU LIKE TO SUPER SIZE THAT?

So here we were with one lump, a handful of doctors, and more decisions to make than we really wanted to. We had to make two fairly major decisions pretty quickly.

The first was what the next surgical option was going to be. We had the choice of going straight to a mastectomy or trying a second lumpectomy. We are sure that most of you reading this book are all too familiar with the pros and cons of each so we will not go into great detail about either.

A mastectomy, single or double, was only necessary if the tumor could not be cleared out of the breast tissue without taking the whole breast. The original tumor was very small and we were able to clear it out with the first lumpectomy. The problem was that Jen had two different types of cancer. One was the invasive carcinoma (that was the original lump that we found) that was easily cleared out at the first surgery. The second was Ductile Carcinoma In Situ (DCIS). This type of breast cancer is much less harmful physically but is much more difficult to clear out of the breast tissue. With a second lumpectomy, we could try to clear out the DCIS and hope for the best. If we did not get clear margins, we could always fall back on the mastectomy. Also, we still needed to have the lymph node biopsy done to discern whether the lymph nodes were positive for cancer or not. Doing this at the lumpectomy would allow us to make some better decisions about things if we had to go the mastectomy route. We consulted with our doctors and surgeons and everybody felt that taking a shot at clearing the margins with a second lumpectomy was well worth the effort.

The other decision to make was about the chemotherapy treatment. This was the only decision that was made during the process that we really did not have all that much input into. It came down to her age, the diagnosis type, whether the lymph nodes were positive or not, and a few other things. It was decided that Jen would receive Adriamycin and Cytoxin for 4 rounds of chemotherapy. She would get treatment once every 21 days.

We went ahead with the second lumpectomy and waited for the results. For the lymph nodes, they needed to do some radio-label dye injections into Jen's nipple so that they could find the appropriate lymph nodes to dissect and check based on which ones were draining fluid from that breast. They were able to do frozen section pathology during surgery and tell us that she was lymph node negative. That was pretty much the first good news we had gotten in this whole process. Jen said that the injections hurt like hell but were worth it in the end. Unfortunately, we got back the rest of the pathology report and found out that the margins were still positive for the DCIS. We would definitely have to go forward with a mastectomy.

Because of the amount of time that had elapsed during the two surgeries, it was agreed that Jen should go into chemotherapy immediately and then have the mastectomy following chemotherapy. We will talk about the Technicolor Rainbow of sights and sounds that was chemotherapy in another chapter.

We now knew that we would have to have at least a single mastectomy done. We started looking much more seriously at the various options for reconstruction and the differences between a single or double mastectomy.

We started looking at the percentage of reoccurrence and how much it grows over time. The odds of Jen having breast cancer again if we went with a single were scary by the time she approached the age at which most women were dealing with it for the first time. We also had some tests done and found a strange area on her other breast. It was not cancerous but was considered abnormal. We thought about it a lot and felt that it was much easier to do this while we were young and did not want to have to do this again in 15 years. Plus we did not want to be scared of every lump and shadow that we found on her other breast. We also took into account the reconstruction option that we had chosen. We were advised that it was better to do both for what we wanted because it would look more symmetrical and less obvious if both were the same. For these reasons, we choose to go with a double mastectomy.

The reconstruction options for a double mastectomy came down to three main options: no reconstruction, Tram-Flap, or implants. No reconstruction was not an option that we seriously considered. If you were really small chested to start with, old enough that it was not worth it to go through the extra surgery and pain, or just plain did not want them, sure don't do it. But Jen wanted to look normal again to herself. And for both of us, we really like her breasts both the old and new versions. We understand why some people would go the no reconstruction or Tram-Flap routes but it was not for us.

The Tram-Flap procedure is where they basically give you a tummy tuck after they remove your breast tissue. They use the tissue from the tummy tuck to build the new breasts. One quick side-note. Technically, these would now be called breast mounds because the actual biological breast tissue is gone. For the purposes of this book, we are going to call them breasts. We understand the difference so please do not correct us if you see us on the street. We just think it sounds stupid, like you are talking about something aliens make in a cornfield or a candy bar. Now back to our breasts. This tissue transfer can be done several different ways using muscle tissue, fat tissue, by total removal of the tissue and reattaching it, or by flipping it under the skin and attaching it to its' original blood supply and muscle and fat can be taken from the abdomen or back.

The big bonus of the Tram-Flap are that it

is all your tissue, no additives and no preservatives. It will feel like your tissue and will move like your tissue. It also can grow and shrink like your normal breasts would as you gain and lose weight. If you happen to be overweight, it would be a bonus tummy tuck. The big downer of it is that you gain a hip to hip belly scar along with doubling your pain and recovery time. One of the other problems that we had with this procedure was that Jen did not have a big enough belly to make breasts of the same size as she had before the mastectomy.

For implants, you have the option of saline and silicone implants. Silicone implants are not approved for cosmetic uses but are for cancer patients. Supposedly, they look and feel more real than do saline implants. The implants would have to be put under the pectoralis muscle which would need to be stretched first. This is done by putting in deflated tissue expanders at the time of the mastectomy. Then, a couple months after the surgery, when the site has healed, the expanders are filled with saline over a period of several months. Once the chosen size has been reached, the expanders are taken out and the permanent implants are put in place.

Implants were the option that we decided to go with, mainly because of the additional scarring, pain, and recovery that would have been induced by the Tram-Flap procedure. Also, we did not want to weaken the abdominal muscles because we wanted to have kids later on. We felt that having it be all natural Jen was not so important in our case as was having her bedridden for an additional two months. We chose saline over silicone because of the additional safety factor of the saline. If it popped, so what? And in truth, neither of us could really feel the difference while holding the implants options in our hands.

I would like to say a few things here about the various surgical options out there at all stages of the process. To reiterate, if you find something and it turns out to be a solid lump, get it taken out of you! A lot of people we have spoken with have told us that they had a hard time convincing their doctors to treat it as potential cancer and to get it taken out. They were told "you are too young to worry about it" and "we see this all the time and it is rarely cancer". The second statement is almost true. But if it turns out to be cancer, and it does sometimes, it makes all the difference to get it early.

When it comes time to check the lymph nodes, surgically, ask for as minimal a procedure as they can do to start rather than going ahead and pulling all of them out. Jen had to have 3 lymph nodes taken out, that's all. The more you take out, the more potential problems you have later in swelling (lymphedema).

The last thing is that we really recommend reading a couple of different books and seeing several different doctors and surgeons. Each of them does things differently whether greatly or slightly. Particularly when it comes to how much skin they take off during the mastectomy, how big the scars are, and where they are going to be. We saw some huge differences in the results (as shown to us by their before and after pictures) among the various surgeons that we went to see. Not that one scarred people worse than others but more in where the scars were located.

So after she had the mastectomy, she was pretty busted up for several weeks. Listen folks, at this point in the process, you are going to see some gruesome things. Even when it goes well, there is a lot of blood and secretions. And the incisions look like a bad knife fight. Suck it up. Don't let her see you cringe or there will be lots of extra crying in your already expanded sea of tears. Also, her mobility is going to be limited so if you can set her up somewhere where she can get around easily on one floor, or in one room most of the time, it would be easier for you both. We bought a recliner so that she could sit up or lay back and nap at her own choice. We also had a bathroom and fridge close by so that if I had to leave her for a bit, she could get a drink and pee. We had home phones with intercom capability. She could page me in the house from where ever she was and actually talk to me so that I did have to go see her to find out what she wants only to find out it was right next to me where I was at before.

The tissue expanders were filled starting about 6 weeks after surgery. This was an extremely painful process. Jen was in more pain from this than she was from the mastectomy itself. Invest in soft moldable ice packs to help with the pain during the expansion process. They sell them at sporting goods stores. It took 3 expansions for us and then we waited a month prior to doing the final implant surgery. During that surgery, Dr. Plastics tried to make the nipples when he was done using the scar tissue from the mastectomy. By 1 month post surgery, you really could barely tell that she had ever had any kind of surgery done on either breast. It was incredible. The area right where the nipples were at prior to all the surgeries there was kind of a flat scar but that was all there was to it. Again, I have got to say wow. It was a lot better than we really expected from seeing all of the gnarly pictures from other plastic surgeons. On a scale of 100 better. Once the tattoos were done, you could not even really tell there had been anything done other than she had fake boobs. There was no mastectomy line like every other person we have seen has nor were there any other scars.

I would love to see doctors show what each of their surgeries look like 2 weeks post op and 6 weeks post op and 1 year post op. I don't think it is easy to visualize the differences and I could not have imagined it looking so good when I think back on the horrible pictures that we saw in some other doctor offices.

After 2 years of post chemotherapy treatment where she took a pill everyday and got a big shot in her stomach every month, my wife was done with her treatment for awhile.

Ideally in our oncologists mind, she would have continued her pills for 3 more years but we wanted to go back to trying for babies again. More on that later.

The last bit of reconstruction that needed to be done was to take another shot at building her nipples. The nipples that the surgeons tried to build during the implant procedure ended up not taking shape the way we wanted, so about eighteen months after that surgery she had the nipples done separately. They told us that might happen so we knew it was going to need to be dealt with at some point. This part was also a little bit painful but not really by comparison of all of the other pains that she had endured. Her biggest issue was that she had to now think about the tops that she wore because the nipples showed in some of them. They were constantly erect so it looked like she was always happy to see you. The nipples were also large because the shrink as they heal. A truly nice problem to have after all the things we had dealt with in the last few years.

After the new additions had healed, we needed to get them tattooed for coloration. I told her to just get a sunburst on one side and a moonburst on the other at the local tattoo shop. She felt that was not the way to go. About a month before we were ready to have this done, her insurance decided to stop dealing with the ENTIRE hospital system where she had all of her surgeries and which housed her plastic surgeon. Yeah, that was a nice petty little stunt on their part.

So we ended up finding another plastic surgeon, one of the ones we had seen in the beginning of it all and asked him to do the tattoos. We went in and he colored them up nicely with some shadowing and everything. I swear after they healed that you would never realize it was all "aftermarket". The tattooing actually makes the nipples appear like that are protruding more than they really are.

This final addition helped my wife's confidence by a factor of 10. She wears more low cut tops than she ever did before and I am constantly telling her that a boob is about to jump out or that she is wearing something inappropriate for the occasion. She never listens to me but that has not changed in our many years together.

One last plug for seriously looking at multiple surgeons. I have seen a lot of other women's pictures and I have yet to see anything as well done as my wife's final product. I have seen many that looked better than I thought they would but a lot that looked so much worse than they had to. Especially if you are a young couple but really for every woman, you have the right to still feel sexy and confident after all of it. A good plastic surgeon is the best way I have seen to do

that. Don't settle for the ones that just try
to save your life today. Expect them to
help save your life both physically and
mentally forever.

7 HUSBANDS TO THE LEFT

I would like to talk about being a husband through all of this. I understand how hard this has been on my wife both mentally and physically. I am willing to propose that I have been there for more of the ugly stuff and cared more for my wife myself than a lot of husbands have in all of this. I am not saying I am the king of husbands by any means and I personally salute any guy who has made it through this with his marriage and sanity intact. I have a great job that is flexible about me working from home and had many weeks of leave banked when this happened. I understand that not everybody is in that situation and maybe can't take time off to go to every appointment. The wonderful thing is that my wife has not bought into the idea that I am not to be involved or treated as a second class citizen in the process as she has been led to believe over and over by the entire breast cancer community.

One of the first things that we noticed when we started down this road was that

many of the women who were in the
doctors' offices were not there with their
husbands. Most were there with their
mothers or a friend or by themselves. We
thought that was really strange. Not
strange like "look at the single women
who have no man to be here with them",
but women who had wedding rings on or
we talked to and know had husbands but
they just weren't ever there. Then we
were given a tour at the cancer center by
one of the support group/therapy staffers.
She gave us a list of all of the support
groups and there was not a single group
for couples or husbands. Seriously, one
of the leading hospitals and clinics in the
country had no support groups for couples
going through one of the most prevalent,
dangerous, and mentally crushing battles
in the medical world. We started
checking around and found that to be true
pretty much across the board. Jen got all
kinds of mail, phone calls, and e-mails
about various support groups, conference
calls, conferences, etc. Not a single one
mentioned husbands. In fact, a couple of
them that "we" wanted to go to, "I", the
one with the penis, was not allowed to go
at all. Mothers, sisters, female friends,

life partners of the same sex.....all of the people could go to the meeting but not the husband.

That shit was strange. I mean, seriously, who would have thought that no such thing existed or that you would be unwelcome to come and hear about what your wife was going through? The answer we got was that women were there to talk about difficult things and innermost feelings and would not want to do that with men around. O.K. I more or less find that credible although, I cannot vouch for your wife, but all mine seems to want to do when I am around is talk about innermost feelings. So then if the women have these inner fears and that deserves a private session.......follow me here...we are about to do some higher math.........wouldn't the husbands or couples have the same need and shouldn't they be given the same support? If one woman wanted to hear what other women in the same situation was doing....again follow closely......wouldn't husbands

want to do the same thing? Or couples,
particularly young couples want to see
what other young couples thought?   What
options they had heard about? Or would
they be willing to show us what their
scars looked like? I mean, you are
making decisions that will affect the rest
of your life in a multitude of ways but
there is nobody to talk to about it. I mean
shit, if I want to buy a house there is a
support group for it and even one for
people that play too many video games.

I just want to take a quick second and note
that I use the word "husband" in this book
because…well….I am a husband. I have
seen a few websites with discussion
groups for caregivers. According to the
definition that we were given, this
included partners and family members as
well as husbands. As much as I feel for
those other two groups and believe that
they have their own story to tell….it is not
my story or Jen's story. So I use husband.
No offense to anyone but the book is
about us. And while I consider Jen my
partner in everything I do and during this
process I have been her caregiver, I am

first, foremost, and most importantly will still be after this is over, her husband.

So I thought I would toss out some things that I thought we might talk about if we were allowed to be a part of a support group. Things like:

How do I deal with working full time and caring for my wife?

Should I tell people at work so they don't think I am just slacking?

How do I deal with family and friends who want to help?

Will this stress change our relationship or ruin it?

Am I allowed to and supposed to have opinions in all of this?

Do I tell my wife what I am thinking and feeling?

What are her breasts going to look like

when this is over?

Will we still be able to have children?

Should I let her sit on the couch or make her get up and get out of the house?

Does anybody know a trick to help her move better when she can't use her arms after surgery?

What do we tell the kids (if you have kids already)?

When do we tell other people?

The list could go on and on. So let's go through that list and I can give you my thoughts on them.

How do I deal with working full time and caring for my wife?

One of the hard things about being the husband in this situation is that you do not get to go on short term disability during this process. Depending on what you do for a living, you may not be able to spend the time with your wife that you want to.

You may not be able to get time off for appointments and surgeries. I was lucky enough to have a ton of leave saved up before this started and have a very understanding and supportive workplace that allowed me to take the time I needed to handle the things in my life. I deeply appreciate that and it reminded me that it is the type of company that I always wanted to work for. Jen's job was the same way. Just all around very supportive of everything. We know we were lucky in this respect. If you do not have this kind of support and flexibility, pick your involvement carefully. Try to attend the appointments in which doctors are discussing treatment plans and test results. If you cannot be there, help her line up someone else to be there with her. These can be really long days, even if it is one appointment. And each time can be different. You can have the same day planned (let's say see doctor at 11 am and treatment at 1 pm) that can be anything from a 4 hour day to a 10 hour day depending on how fast or slow the clinics are moving that day. It sucks to be sitting there all day by yourself.

Should I tell people at work so they don't think I am just slacking?

I chose to tell selected coworkers and of course my bosses so that they knew where I was and how to find me during this time. I did not broadcast it but word travels fast and most people knew what was going on. I work for a pretty close knit company and had worked with many of the people for years so they tried their best to cover for me and went out of their way to not bother me when I was not at the office.

How do I deal with family and friends who want to help?

Getting more help than needed was very difficult for me to handle. I realize that it is probably more likely that most of you are not getting help when you need it if you have kids or a job that won't let you off. My issue is that I am a huge control freak. I mean off the charts. Someone coming in and doing my laundry is just mindboggling for me to handle. I know that most people would love that to happen but not me. First, I take it as an insult that I cannot take care of my wife and myself or that I cannot cook for her or clean my own house. I know that it is not meant that way. I really do, honest. But I just would rather do things myself. I also understand that sometimes other people need to help us to help them deal with the situation better. So I tried to let that happen. I…uh…..probably did not always succeed with that. Looking back now, I realize that if you find things for others to do to help, it lets them feel better and it is one less thing you have to do.

Now, don't get me wrong. There were times we needed help. There were a few days that I had to be at work because of a client visit or a deadline and needed somebody to do something for Jen. And I am very grateful for having my parents close by, a mother-in-law and two brother-in-laws (and sister-in-law) who would drop everything and come down anytime we asked and lots of friends who were able to do things for us.

Will this stress change our relationship or ruin it?

This is discussed in other chapters.

Am I allowed to and supposed to have opinions in all of this?

Every husband, if he loves his wife, has to be scared in this process. Personally, my greatest fear has always been losing my wife, even before I had one. I think I saw some crappy made for TV movie as a kid where the mom died in child birth and the dad had to raise a little girl by himself. Ever since then, it has scared me to death. Jen was sick and scared enough that I tried very hard not to burden her with my fears. We talked about them some and I leaned heavily on Jen's brothers, who are as close as brothers to me, and my friends. But I have to admit that it would have been nice to talk to other men that were going through this. Total strangers maybe but men who were in the same situation. Women have made a whole sorority out of it and as soon as you say "I have breast cancer" they recite a lineage of everybody they have ever known who has had it and

give you their numbers to call them and talk. Hell, Lifetime has made practically a whole network on programming based on it. I have rarely talked to a husband who has had a wife with breast cancer. They are like Big-foot...you wouldn't even know one existed but you see blurry pictures once in awhile. I have found a few online and conversed with some more than others. The ones that I have talked to have given much the same feedback as I have felt. A few are just starting the process and I have been able to offer them some insight and advice that has helped them through parts. Imagine if we were able to put a bunch of us in a room to talk about things? I think we could do a lot of good for ourselves and for future couples. If you want to stop drinking you get a Sponsor who you can call for advice or to talk to when you are struggling.
Wouldn't it be helpful as hell to have the same system for breast cancer? For both the husbands and wives?

I figure some guys have to work or some

are just squeamish. But I cannot fathom
why you would not want to be there with
your wife. I highly encourage you to be a
part of this process. If you are reading
this, you probably are trying to be already.
But keep on being there. This may be a
long term issue that you have to deal with.
Your wife may be under anesthesia or out
of it and you have to answer the questions
and make the decisions. You can't do that
very well if you have not been on board
from the beginning.

One advantage I had in this is that I, as
does Jen, do biomedical research. We
knew what the doctors were talking about.
We could read the pathology reports
pretty well and knew what they meant.
We had worked with many of the drugs
that she was prescribed. I could not
imagine going through this if we were
both in other professions.

If you find yourself in this situation, do
the research. Don't believe everything
that you read or hear but read enough that
you at least are familiar with the terms

that are being tossed at you in doctors' visits. When you are told about a drug or procedure, research it and write down questions if you have them. Jen and I go to almost every appointment with a list of questions to ask.

The blow that cancer deals to the sex life of a couple is a big enough issue that I put that in a separate chapter. But I think that many men are uncertain if sex is even something they should ask about or talk about. You can and you should. It won't make me popular with the women's groups or Oprah but it is (can be anyway) a big part of a marriage and when totally taken away, it has some obvious effects on both parties.

Do I tell my wife what I am thinking and feeling?

Yes, you cannot hold it inside you the whole time. It is not good for you and will not be good for your marriage. You may have to pick a time to share your feelings that is appropriate but you should really try to talk to her as much as you can.

What are her breasts going to look like when this is over?

This is really variable and will depend totally on what surgical option you choose to have done. We have seen some extremely different outcomes. My wife's breasts are spectacular and you have to know what you are looking for to realize that it is all not real.

Will we still be able to have children?

This will depend on each person and you should talk to you Oncologist about this if that is an important issue for you as a couple. It may be that it is still a viable option down the line or it may be that it is not. But you should ask what the odds are in your case. For us, fertility was a HUGE issue.

Should I let her sit on the couch or make her get up and get out of the house?

I will discuss this in detail in another chapter. You have to pick your battles but sitting in the dark watching Lifetime and WE TV doesn't help anyone.

Does anybody know a trick to help her move better when she can't use her arms after surgery?

This will be talked about in another chapter. Get creative.

What do we tell the kids (if you have kids already)?

This was not applicable for us. But there are books to help explain it to your kids and many cancer centers offer a seminar that you can take young children to that helps them talk about it.

When do we tell other people?

I cover this in detail in later chapters. I would say to embrace it and not hide it. People find out eventually.

8 I THINK MY VIRGINITY IS GROWING BACK

One of the biggest things that we have discovered that nobody talks about when you are going through breast cancer treatment is the effect that it all has on the sex life of the couple in question.

Jen was being poked and prodded by all kinds of people and the most nakedness I was seeing was at doctor's appointments. Seriously, it was like Girls Gone Wild there was so much breastage. By the way, why did doctors leave the room while Jen took off her shirt, but then she took off the little robe once they came back in? I do not understand that one at all. Anyway, Jen has been either sore from surgery or tissue expanders, sick from chemotherapy, or suffering from forced chemically induced menopausal side effects for the better part of 12 months as I started writing this book and as I finish it, we are going on 9 years. That is a long time but not nearly as long as it can be for some couples where the wife has to go through much more chemotherapy, radiation, or post-chemo Tamoxifen than Jen has received.

The first reaction that most people have is probably going to be "well your wife is sick, she is vomiting, and losing her womanhoodness, so the least you can do is not bug her about sex, you little pervert". Well, that is pretty much true. It also relays the theme that permeates all of the breast cancer phenomenon, which is that the husbands barely exist and are not going through this, just the wife is. Which is bull shit. It also ignores the fact that most women have a sex drive of their own that they are probably missing out on just as much as the husband.

You would be right to say that it is pretty acceptable for her not to be in the mood. Honestly, even as a man, I was not in the mood as much as I would normally be. Which I will be honest and say is most of the time normally. But it still happens on both sides. We had a very healthy and active sex life prior to this. I will freely admit that I, at 30+, have the sex drive of a 16 year old. I just can't help it. My wife is gorgeous, and I just cannot keep my hands off of her. I apologize to Jen's brothers, who probably just dropped the book and ran to the bathroom to vomit, but that is just how it is. By the way, if you know us personally and don't want to hear any further details of our sex life, you might want to skip the rest of this chapter.

So we have found ways to get the job done for both of us, as needed. We bought a lot of porn the past few years. We did this both for me and also so that we could play together when Jen was not feeling well enough to have sex with me but needed some attention in what we now refer to as "Area 51". We took a lot of extra time to make out and fool around that we did not always do prior to sex after 5 years of marriage.

We had to pick our spots carefully for when we wanted to have sex. It was generally only once every 3 or 4 weeks,

which may seem like a lot to some
married guys out there but was hard to get
used to when we were used to 2-3 times a
week. We usually would talk about it at
dinner and found that it was easier if we
went to bed earlier that night and then I
would be even more attentive physically
to her that evening than I normally am.
We sit next to each other and hold hands
or cuddle when we watch TV normally
but I would make a special effort to
convince her body to cooperate. We
purchased special lubes to help out as
well. We found certain positions that
made it more comfortable for her or
increased her pleasure that were different
from normal. We found that using other
stimulation in conjunction with sex helped
Jen out a lot.

I do not intend this to be terribly graphic
but the point is that you need to try to
have a marriage even though your wife
has breast cancer. If you normally have
sex as a part of your marriage,
well..........

As the husband, you need to talk about this with your wife. If she is not interested and does not want to work with you on it, go in the bathroom like you have since age 13 and handle your business so that it does not bother her. I know it is not very sexy but I always asked Jen if she was interested before I did anything else. She might be intending to sneak attack me when I got to bed because she felt good that day. But if I just got rid of the Evils and went to bed without knowing....well then there was lots of crying. Plus, and you would have to ask Jen about this, but I think it helped her mentally that I still found her attractive and sexy. That I still wanted her, even if she was bald and had acquired a few new scars.

You cannot give her the support she needs and handle the stress in the process without some kind of relief or release. If sex is that release for you, or for both of you, try to keep doing it when you can. If it is not but golf is...well you are kind of

weird but hey dude, go play golf. My
general point is that you need to take care
of not only the wife going through surgery
and chemo and her physical needs from
those issues but also you need to take care
of your marriage and of each other. If
making love gently makes you both
happy, try to keep doing that when you
can. On the other hand, if you don't
normally have sex much…..well…..sadly
it may not be an issue for you. Plus you
have that golf thing you like so much.

In general, I just wanted to put it out there
for other men to realize that they are not
the only ones who might think about it.
Obviously, there may be physical
limitations. One of the reasons it was
important to me was that at that point, I
had never felt that Jen was going to die.
Yeah, a panic attack here or there and it
may have crossed my mind but at no point
in the process did I truly allow myself to
think that she was going to die on me. So
I looked at it as something we had to go
through but I always tried to think about
the long term health of our marriage and
our relationship. I did not want to make it

through this only to have no marriage left afterwards. So much for the sex talk.

9 CLEAN UP ON AISLE 3!

If you are like we were at the time…under 30…no kids…….and the dogs are house trained, you probably are used to living a more or less secretion free lifestyle. That my friend….is about to change. It's all about the Secretions, baby!

Again, my wife and I do research and so we are used to wearing gloves and handling bloody gauze. It helps not to be squeamish in the process. But Wow. The things chemotherapy does to the body……Wow. My wife essentially turned in a human secretion piñata. Except that you did not have to hit her with a cut off broomstick.

It was extremely hard on me to see my wife in pain and not to be able to kick someone's ass or yell at them for causing it. Being a control freak, I am very "fix the problem" oriented. But there is really nothing you can do about it. The big things that you are responsible for is taking care of her when she is down. Remember the "in sickness and in health" part?

I struggled walking the fine line between allowing Jen to feel down on herself and in pain when she needed to and in pushing her to be up and about when she could be. This was both during chemo and also for her surgeries. I got yelled at for making her get up or leave the house sometimes but if I had let her just lay there, it would have been so much worse for her emotionally and allowed her to sink further into a depressed state.

Although we received all kinds of stuff in the mail from people, there is really not much that we needed to buy or receive that could have helped during the process. I think having a recliner, which we bought shortly after diagnosis, really helped a lot because she could be "up" and downstairs

with the family (me, the dogs, and
whoever was there that weekend) without
having to truly sit up. The other item that
helped was that our cordless phones had
an intercom system so that she could call
me and ask for something specific without
me going to where she was and then
going back to get what she wanted.

There are a few other things that would be
a good idea to keep around:

A water tight trash can or bucket for
projectile vomiting. Maybe a couple of
them placed in any room she might hang
out in during the day.

Lots of extra soft and absorbent towels. I
mean lots. If you think you have enough,
buy 4 more.

A small handheld carpet cleaner. They
cost about $30 and will help save carpets
from needing replacing when the process

is over.

Put carpeting or a large bath carpet in the bathroom she will be using. Gives some cushioning during vomiting.

Cases of bottled water. Even if you normally drink tap water, having ready water that can be dropped, knocked over, put in a bag, or tucked next to her on the bed or chair, is really useful.

Make up or buy bags of crushed ice. Useful for everything from chewing when she can't eat anything else…. to using in icepacks because they conform better than cubes.

Gel ice packs from a sporting goods store. You can't have enough.

Try to set up an area that she can be in with everything in easy access. For example, we had a recliner and set up a side table where she could keep a phone, drinks, snacks, etc. in easy reach. And it was right next to a bathroom.

Whatever her safety food is, you want to try to identify this early in the struggle. In Jen's case it was Won Ton soup broth and Ramen noodles. She could almost always keep that down. Plus, if she does decide to hurl them at you like a split tonsil fastball, they came up easily and did not rip her esophagus up on the ride. On the flip side of that, never try to make her favorite (pre-chemo) meal during this. I know it sounds nice of you to make her that special dish but if she hurls it, she will dislike the item forever after it's all over.

Extra sheets and pillows. Some things, pillows especially, are easier to replace than to clean.

We tried to have a routine that we followed each time she had a treatment. Again, yours will have to be made up by you based on her schedule and what works with her body. Ours was to eat at the same restaurant after the treatment because she could eat that night without being sick until the next day. She was able to get one last good solid meal in before she turned into the human volcano.

Now there were also a bunch of different drugs that she was given to try to alleviate these side effects. Ummm…yeah…some of those are not so good. From what we heard, they affect each person differently and they try them until they find one that works for you. Good idea in theory but the first set she got made her violently ill. After that, the ones she took helped some but she was by no means normal. They will most likely give you a list of foods to avoid and things to try to help her. In our experience, it seems to be different for each person so feel free to do something that is not on the list.

Your job now and for the rest of her treatment schedule is to try to make her comfortable and do whatever you can to get her to eat, stay hydrated, and sleep as much as possible.

One of the things that we did that was extremely useful was to have a two comforter system in the bed. We had a light comforter under a heavy comforter. This allowed her to choose from three different levels of warmth during the night. The chemotherapy really jacked up her ability to thermoregulate and keeping her warm or cool enough was a constant battle. Now, I did spend time every night and morning fixing the blankets since she would kick them into disarray every night but in general it helped a lot.

This heat issue manifests itself in all aspects of the day so be ready with an array of blankets around the house and jackets of various weights in the car. Many times my lovely wife would call me a bad name because I asked her if she wanted a jacket to go out while she was dripping in sweat only to have her ask for that jacket 20 minutes later. If it is chilly enough that you are taking a jacket, take her one. If not, you will lose yours in route. Heat can be controlled also through proper use of socks and hats. Again, it can sometimes be a pain but just grab a hat and put it in your pocket. Jen did not wear wigs too often (thankfully because they scared the dogs and I thought they were freaky) so she wore hats and scarves most of the time willfully.

If her drugs have to be given every 4 to 6 hours, set your alarm for the middle of the night and get up to give her the medications. If it waits until morning, you will both regret it. Believe me, we are not morning people and I hate to wake up in the middle of the night but it needed to be done. You do not want to get behind the timeline here. Once nausea sets in, it is hard to keep the pills down and then if she yacks one up it is all over. Get one of those pill boxes and put whatever she needs each time in there. Then you just get up, whip out the pills from a single place, and hand her a bottle of water.

Feed her anytime she asks and then turn around and ask her if she wants to eat as often as you can. She most likely will not be able to eat much at any given time but she might be able to eat a bunch of small meals over the course of the day. We kept a lot of little things like applesauce and fruit around for her to eat and then I would make things that could be made then put in the refrigerator and heated up the next time she wanted some later that day.

Side Note here…we had some people get us this personal chef person who made meals then dropped them off. This is one of those things that sounds great on paper but are not as helpful as you would think. These things are generally yuppie gourmet meals which taste great if you like rosemary and pine nuts but are probably too weird or spiced for her to handle on a bad stomach. Again, great idea but may be more helpful the first week she goes back to work.

Back to feeding. Whatever you can get her to eat, let her eat it. True, 6 cases of Ramen noodles over 4 months are not exactly the Surgeon Generals diet plan but whatever you can do to keep food moving through her system in the correct direction and without making a U-Turn, is worthwhile. You can get the nutritious stuff into her later.

Cleaning up after she has made a mess of some area is not always easy to do. To be honest, our dogs puke in the toilet (dead serious) so I am not big on the random bodily secretions in the middle of the night. But it happens. From all sorts of areas. The two keys to the game plan on this one are to make sure you have everything you need close at hand and to make it happen as quickly as possible.

I tried to have a set of sheets, a pillow, a change of clothes, and a blanket ready to go so that I could just rip it all off and replace it in about 2 minutes. She was

usually crying and apologizing at this
point so the less time it takes to get her
comfortable and back in bed, the better.
The other upside of doing this is that if
you clean her up and get her back in bed,
you can then go throw the items in the
wash or trash as needed and get back into
bed quickly yourself. Less disruption for
both of you. Plus, the majority of the time
she did not remember yakking by next
morning so she was less upset the next
day if there was nothing making her
remember it. I tried not to mention it
unless she brought it up or asked if she
did because it always upset her to make a
mess. Another useful thing here is a
waterproof mattress cover. Like you have
for kids. Or if you are a big sweaty guy
or your wife is sick. This saved our
mattress, and made clean up easier as
well. You can also try layering sheets by
having a set on the bed, under the current
set and protected by a towel or something.
Your other option is to just pull things off
the bed or take the now soiled trashcan
into the bathroom and leave it until
morning. Your call.

The last thing I would like to talk about to prepare you for is the gas. Gentlemen, I don't know anything about you but if you are a guy, you fart. Period, don't try to hide it. It probably smells bad most of time. I am proud to say that I can clear my dogs out of the whole top floor of the house when I get a good one. The same dogs that roll in dead things because they think it's sexy.

Dude, I got nothing on my wife once the chemo started up. Chemo by definition is killing off all of the fast growing cells in your body. Among these were her intestinal lining. Dear god, it makes for a horrid stench. Seriously, I cried a few times and begged for mercy. It was not her fault and she was very embarrassed by it. But there was nothing she could do. It would just come busting out.

But here is the good news! Again, being men, you most likely have a couple of farts on deck all the time and an ability to fire them off at will. This is normally something that disgusts and reviles my wife but during chemotherapy....I am like a superhero with a mutant power. You remember sitting in class or the movies and you lean over to your buddy and say "dude, on 3 cough, O.K.?" Your buddy knew what that meant and 5 guys could pull this off with the precision timing of Navy Seals. Well, this skill was now put to use by my wife, who would lean over and request that I fire off a practice round to cover her so that everybody would think the smell came from me. Being proud of my intestinal fortitude as I am, I was even more proud to take credit for the salvo of Napalm that she was throwing out there. We became the stinky version of the Wonder Twins.

10 MENOPAUSE BLOWS

The diagnosis of your wife having breast cancer is going to change your life forever. It is most likely going to change it several times in vastly different directions. Do not think for one second that it is going to be a situation where she has a surgery and then a little bit of chemotherapy and then you roll right back into your old life. It is a very long process even in the best case scenarios. Be ready for that and plan accordingly.

Jen and I have some very good communication skills with each other and we really understood that this was going to be a long term process. We came up with a plan for what we wanted to see happen and structured our lives around that plan.

So she had surgery after surgery. Then she had chemotherapy. After the chemotherapy came Jen's double mastectomy. Then came tissue expanders

and the inflation of the implants and then
those had to be removed and have the
permanent ones put into place. This was
followed by Tamoxifen and injections
which sent her into an early menopause.
And that's where the fun really began.

Most of us probably lived through or are
in the process of living through our
mothers going through menopause. If you
are reading this as a fairly young husband
of a young wife, most likely you were not
planning on worrying about your wife
doing any menopause related activities for
a good long time. Well, here comes the
next round of indignities.

Let me say that Jen having to go through
surgeries sucked. As did chemotherapy.
But I really think that the menopause
portion of the show was almost as bad as
the chemotherapy. The chemo only made
her sick for a few months and it was only
really bad for about a week out of each
round. But the menopause thing…..that
sucks for two to five years. Every day.
Round the clock.

Let's start off by talking about the

crying......oh the crying. My loving wife got hit by the hormone train pretty quickly once the post-chemotherapy treatment started. It is basically designed to rip every drop of Estrogen out of the woman's body so that the ER+ breast cancer that is essentially living off of the Estrogen has no food and therefore dies off.   If there is anything left to begin with after chemo. Hold on...we need to review that part again to make sure that everybody understood....the womanly body which has heretofore been pumping out tons of Estrogen every day since they were 12 years old is now running on empty.

This, my friends, is what we call a "bad situation for everybody". You know how the women folk get a *little emotional*, sometimes, around their period? On occasion there might be *some* random crying, screaming, or *mild* moodiness in a few women at the least (wink wink nudge nudge). Well that is because they were getting surges of that same hormone. Let me clue you in to a little secret…that shit works in both directions. When you all of a sudden take away that lovely little hormone.....bad things happen.

My wife is a little bit emotional on a normal day (sorry Sweetness) and has been known to start crying for a sundry of reasons that I never would consider crying about. But she was playing on a different level once these drugs hit her system. She began to cry on a many times a day basis. Over anything you can imagine. Legitimate reasons such as "I have cancer", "I am bald", "I had a mastectomy", and others became daily players in the "why I was crying" show. But the guest spots come from places like "where are my shoes, I can't find my shoes", "I just farted in public", and my personal favorite "I am so tired I can't sleep". So be ready for there to be lots of crying.

This is another of many reasons why there are stations on cable such as "E", Lifetime, Lifetime movies, and ABC family. At one point that year, I used the parental controls on our TV to block out all of these stations because I would come home everyday to find my wife crying while watching Meredith Baxter Burney in yet another Made for TV "Based on a True Story" movie about somebody dying or being eaten by wolves. Why do they put that stuff on there? Do any married guys work at those stations? If you happen to be reading this and you are a married guy who works at Lifetime, please tell them to stop it. Nobody wins except Puffs and Hagen Das.

It became a problem for her emotional state so I blocked it out. Unfortunately, I did not tell her I was doing so and when I came home the next day, she was laying on the floor with the remote control crying like a Crack addict because she could not watch the episode of some horrible Lifetime network show that she wanted so desperately to watch. So we negotiated a truce involving supervised viewing of these channels and no

Meredith Baxter Burney or Justine
Bateman movies under any
circumstances.

There are many other wonderful little
surprises that are about to come your way
but the biggest of all is the arrival of the
hot flashes. These are about to become
the overriding power in your life until
such time as the treatment is over and
your wife comes out of menopause which
in some cases may not happen.

What is a hot flash? It is when you are
sitting in a perfectly reasonably
temperature room that instantly becomes
the 6th circle of Hell. You turn red and
sweat starts to pour off of your body like
Patrick Ewing at the foul line. In a matter
of minutes you are soaked through your
clothes. Oh yeah, then it goes away and
you're freezing as the sweat evaporates
from your body. Much fun all around.

Most of us, as men, have an innate ability

to thermoregulate that seems to have passed by the females of our species during the evolutionary process. But this is something truly astonishing that would defeat even our abilities to adapt. The arrival of hot flashes presents some new and exciting challenges for her and for you.

One of these challenges involves sleeping. Being young and in love with my wife, prior to cancer, we slept pretty much curled around each other every night. One of us would hold the other and we could easily fit into a twin size bed. We actually sleep in a queen sized bed which means that the dogs have plenty of room to stretch out. Well, with the hot flashes this becomes essentially impossible because at the first sign of a hot flash, I would get kicked and elbowed as she tried to escape into the cold. The dogs learned this rather quickly and gave up sleeping on her side of the bed after about 2 weeks.

I was not that quick on the uptake and garnered several nasty bruises from flying

Michael Streicker

heels and elbows. When she finally badly bloodied my nose in her need to escape my clutches, I gave up. We have a hard sided bed and I have learned to sleep with my body wrapped up on the wooden side as far from the flailing as possible. Since I cannot sleep without touching her I have adapted to placing my palm on the top of her head where she can remove it when she gets hot and but I can put it back when the flash is over. This has worked out well for our sleeping but my rugby teammates do not appreciate it when I do the same to them on road trips. I have learned that it is better to warn them ahead of time.

We talked earlier about the need to have two sets of blankets on the bed to assist your wife in her thermoregulatory endeavors. That will help, however, you are about to play what my wife and I call the "covers game". This entails going to sleep with the covers on BOTH of you equally. Then she gets a hot flash and proceeds to throw off the covers. This can occur in one of two directions....fully on top of you or on the floor. In situation one, fully on top of you, you can either learn to deal with it and sweat heavily yourself or you can move far enough away from her in the bed that there is room for her to deposit the blankets between you for her to get to later. In situation two, on the floor, she will then proceed to take what little bit of covers you might be left holding or attempt to burrow under you to get warm at the end of the hot flash. Remember what I said earlier, once it is over, the sweat evaporates and she will be freezing in short order. My tactics for this were simple. I learned to wrap my end of the blankets under my legs when I went to sleep so that she could not throw them off the other side. I usually still wake up when she attempts to rip the covers off of me before placing them between us but it is less loss of sleep than getting up to put the covers back on the bed 6 times a night.

The other major challenge is going out in public. You have to learn to pack extra clothes that might be needed and also get used to carrying jackets, sweaters, and other pieces of clothing that she starts discarding as she walks through the mall or sits at dinner. Just get in the habit of keeping two or three different jackets, hats, and scarves in the car. I swear it will work out in the end. She has learned to keep extra clothes in her office at work so that she can change if need be in the middle of the day.

11 IS IT COLD IN HERE?

One of the side effects that my wife had from chemotherapy and her post chemo treatment was memory loss. Not just a little bit but like the character from the Adam Sandler movie that only could remember things for 10 seconds. No joke. This was actually the hardest thing for me to get used to of all of the side effects.

The following is a re-cap of the average night in our house:

"Hi honey, how was your day?"

"Good, and you?"

"Good"

2 minutes goes by and then

"How was your day today?"

"Ummmm….fine."

"Aren't you going to ask me how my day was?"

"I already know how it was."

"How do you know that?"

"Because we just had this conversation 2 minutes ago."

"No we didn't."

"Uh..yes we did."

"UH NO WE DID NOT!"

"Yes, dear."

2 minutes goes by and then

"How was your day?"

Seriously…it was bad. I am smarter than the average bear and was able to quickly grasp that this was a side effect and then it became easier for me to understand and not to be as annoyed with this little game. Now, getting Jen to believe me when I told her she did this was a whole different battle. I actually resorted to having her sign a note saying that she had talked to me about something. After 5 or 6 times that I handed her a note saying that we had this conversation, she began to believe me. Just a warning but the temptation to abuse this particular side effect is huge. You can essentially talk your wife into believing that she agreed to all sorts of stuff. Don't do it.

Why you may ask? Because it goes both
ways. Just as she does not remember
having the conversation with you, she also
will argue to the death that she HAD a
conversation with you but you do not
remember it. My working theory is that
she has these conversations in her head or
practices them with the dogs before she
talked to me but her mind convinces her
that the conversation was real. One such
conversation is recapped below.

"Honey, remember to be home by 5 so
that we can go over to Katie's for dinner."

"Ummmm….say what?"

"We are going to Katie and John's for
dinner tonight. We talked about this last
week and you agreed to go."

"Ummm….no we didn't and I agreed to

no such thing. I have hockey tickets tonight so I can't go."

"But you promised me we could go to dinner with them!"

"But I don't like them, I don't ever go out with them."

"But you promised!" (Small tears start to form, which I believe is cheating).

"When exactly did we have this conversation?"

"Saturday morning when we were cuddling in bed."

"Yeah, I was not there. I was at a rugby game Pittsburgh...that was the dog."

I still ended up going to that dinner.

She also had a very hard time remembering what she was doing from minute to minute. She would get up when we were watching a movie and walk upstairs to get a drink and not come back. When I went to find her, she was watching TV in bed or talking on the phone. Or worse, she would come downstairs without a drink and ask me what she went up there for.

Again, your job as the husband is to try to help out and minimize these affects on her daily life. E-mail helps so I send her lots of little reminders about things that she is supposed to do during the day or that night. Also, I try to provide helpful little hints and reminders about things during conversations. This will get you yelled at from time to time. You will hear phrases such as "I'm doing it!" and "I am a grown ass adult, stop checking up on me!". But in the long run, it is better for you both to do it. And she will also occasionally thank you for the help or reminder.

Until this point in our lives, I was in charge of very little of our social calendar. I did not even pretend I was in the know. But now that her memory is suspect, most of these items at least cross my awareness. She is still in charge but I make sure that she has it all in order. We missed a couple of events because I did not know about it and she forgot. So know we just put in on the calendar and I check it once in awhile.

If you do not already do so, I strongly suggest using a shared calendar. With the advent of smart phones, this has become easier as she now has a calendar with her pretty much at all times. She or I can add things and it updates the other person. It helps us to avoid double booking ourselves as well. We have the calendar set up to send us reminder notifications so that things do not get forgotten.

In addition, I highly suggest putting the word out to your friends and family about this little problem so that they tell you about things as well. We have asked that people send as much as they can in the form of e-mail and copy both of us. Your job is make sure that things happen as scheduled. But not everyone feels that it is "necessary" to run things by you, the husband. You may be seen as somehow "controlling" your wife's time but in general, people adapt and get with the program.

12 MANAGING THE PERCEPTION

As you and your wife go through the breast cancer process from diagnosis to treatment to surgery and beyond, you need to decide who is in control of the situation. You and she need to be the decision makers and stay on the same page in all of this. That can be hard because a lot of people are going to pressure you in their own way.

Think about this in terms of a sports team. On any team, you have general managers, coaches, and players. And then you have the fans and sports talk radio. You and your wife are the GM's because you are the ones responsible for hiring the coaches. The coaches are the doctors because they call the plays. You and your wife are also the players because you can choose to call audibles or you can choose free agency and go play for another coach. The fans and sports talk radio callers are all the people around you telling you their opinion about what you should be doing. The one thing that is sure to cause the collapse of any team is when the players, coaches, and GM's start listening to the fans and the callers on sports radio. Don't let that happen.

It is vital that you and your wife decide who (other than the two of you) gets information and when they get it. You have to hold a certain number of press conferences during the process. What we did was develop security levels of a sort. Basically we decided who we wanted to have what level of detailed information. Everybody got the group emails (we talked about those earlier) but some people got a phone call after each treatment. We also had caller ID so a lot of the time, we just did not pick up the phone. In the new world of technology, we have a phone that verbally tells us who is calling and it shows up on our TV screen. We are extremely judicious in our use of the Caller ID.

If someone is bothering you and pushing

for information above their designated security level, then the Designated Asshole comes into play.

In our relationship, I am the Designated Asshole. To those that know me, it will come as no surprise. When we can't do something like go out to dinner with somebody or if we do not want to tell somebody something, it is because "Mike doesn't want to". It is easier for this time period if you are the Designated Asshole because she is sick and it is harder to blame shit on her. Your other option is to say "She does not feel up to it". We did use that one a couple of times. There will be times when people want to come over or want to make you dinner or whatever when you both just want to have a weekend alone or sit in the house. This is when you get to work your magic. It will not improve your personal popularity with those folks but your wife will love you and that is all that matters. Again, it depends on who the people are. We have some friends that we have unfortunately

bailed on at the last minute several times
because Jen was not feeling up to
whatever we were supposed to do that
day. As the years have gone on, we don't
hide this as much as we used to hide it.
Our friends know that a lot of our
activities are tentative based on how she
feels that day. During some parts of her
treatment (on and off for 9 years now), we
have had a really good idea of when it
was safe to plan things. At other points, it
is a daily crap shoot of how she might
feel.

And you are going to need that love for
her to tap into. Why? Because the
Designated Asshole's other job is to push
your wife to keep on fighting. Pretty
much everybody else will be Enablers.
They will tell her to just sit in bed and
relax, or to take as many painkillers as she
needs to, or whatever. Your job is to
manage that and at the same time be able
to kick her out of bed and make her
continue her life as normally as she can
through all of this. Breast cancer is
depressing. It sucks the big one. But
guess what, if you are able to beat it or at

least hold it at bay, you have to still have a life and a marriage to keep going as well. Your job has to be to know when it is the right time to push her a little and when it is the right time to coddle her. There are days that you have to let her lay in bed and do nothing and then there are days you have to make her get up and focus on living her life. At all stages of the process, she will have good days and bad days physically and the same can be said mentally.

As difficult as many other parts of the process are, this is what was truly the hardest thing for me to gauge each day. With everybody else around her giving in and letting her do whatever she wanted and whenever she wanted, you may need to be the gatekeeper of her mental health. Depending on how your wife handles things, she may face serious issues with depression or she may just need some help here and there along the way to keep herself together. The others get to come and go and really never see the bad shit, no matter how much they call or visit. They don't get the fun parts like the wake up in the middle of the night with her crying, the rocking back and forth sobbing. They get to feed her some ice cream and fluff her pillow and go home. It's the equivalent of being an Uncle when you don't have kids of your own. You get to play with them and then go home when they puke. You really have to be careful of letting the depression get to be too severe. There were times I had to literally drag her out of bed, make her shower, and take her to a movie. But you have to find ways to distract her from the depression. I would make her come with me when I was just running errands just to get her out of the house. This can backfire on you if you let her shop when weak and depressed. We now have an extra parakeet because I let her come into the pet store while I was getting dog food. She thought the one we had was bored since he had been getting less attention than he normally did. I know it sounds mean but you will probably have to be the one to decide when she is bordering on going over the edge and pull her back.

During the whole thing, I have tried to do my best to keep her centered on what was really important...her getting through this healthy, physically, and mentally with our marriage intact. Being a young couple going through this, you have some handicaps to deal with that the older couples do not. They have their own set of issues to deal with I suppose but again, this book is about us so I focus on ours.

The biggest one of those handicaps is that we were at the age where society tells you that it is time for you to start cranking out children. We had just started trying a few months prior to her diagnosis and it crushed her to go from trying to have cute little babies to dealing with the possibility that we would not be able to have children. She had just talked me into the trying to have children and she was so happy about it only to have that taken away from her.

I made the mistake early on by telling her

that I did not really care if we had kids, that I married her because I wanted to spend the rest of my life with her. Not because I thought she would make a great mother or because I wanted her to have my children. All that mattered to me was getting her healthy and living many years together. Even if it's just us. Somehow, that was not an appropriate response to the situation because she was all sorts of pissed off at me. So I changed my message to "I really desperately want to have children with you but we cannot right now. But when we can, we will do everything possible to have them together." This seemed to be the right answer in my case. So gauge that one carefully. You may have to change your answer to that a couple of times as you go along. The good thing it that she will likely forget what you said the last time.

Because you are at the "breeding age", you are constantly going to be asked about when you are going to have some kids. It's just part of the small talk that people make at work, dinner parties, and family reunions. Most of the time, even

people who know your situation, know
she is currently going through chemo but
they still ask because it is what they are
programmed to do. And none of them are
doing it to be mean or to rub it in that you
don't have any kids and may not be able
to have any. They just do it because
that's what you do over punch and
cookies. It's like dating for 6 months and
going to your cousin's wedding.
Everybody in the place is going to ask
you "so when are you two going to get
married?" That is just how shit works in
the world. So be ready for it. Have an
answer ready for when it comes up. I
have a couple of them depending on what
mood I am in and if I want to roll with it
or send a message back to the person that
they should not have asked the question.
My answers range from "we are waiting
until her health is better" to "right now
my wife is trying to stay alive so it is sort
of on the back burner". I have a couple of
nastier ones too but I try hard not to use
those.

At the same time, most of the couples you know will be having children. And every single time that happens, your wife will cry. Deep down she is happy for them but she is also mad at the world for her being the only woman (in her mind) who is not having children. As a guy, I do not really have a biological clock. If I do, it's busted. I have some friends that definitely have them and were all about having some kids. I really like to sleep and don't really care for wiping another person's ass, so I have never felt like I was missing all that much. But she will feel that way. Every evolutionary molecule in her body is telling her that has to have children. That she is a failure as a wife and as a woman if she cannot have children. That she is missing out on the love and miracle of life. There are whole cable channels such as Lifetime, Lifetime Movies, and Discovery Health Channel that reinforce this belief. All they show are these great made-up movies about miracle babies or documentaries about the 1 out of 1000 couples that were able to have a baby under the most dire circumstances. They never mention the others and those couples do not have a show to talk about their lives. Because it would not reinforce the right image of happy mothers and babies.

This was really a very slippery slope that you have to handle carefully. We have talked some about the lack of men I have noticed in clinics and with their wives during treatment. Well apparently some of that is because there are a bunch of guys that leave their wives when breast cancer pops up. Jen went out to a lunch with some women and she was one of only two women (out of 8) that the man (husband or boyfriend) had not left them because they got cancer. Their reasons in some cases were an otherwise bad marriage that cancer just put over the edge or because the women might not be able to have kids anymore. One guy left because they only had one kid and he wanted more. O.K., so these guys may or may not be assholes. But in the realm of breast cancer, for some reason, a lot of guys get spooked so be aware that your wife may be extremely sensitive about the subject. She may even give you the "leave me and be with someone else who can give you health and children" speech. Mine did. Several times actually. I started laughing because it was so ridiculous. But be aware of what they might be hearing from other women as they go to support groups that you are not allowed to attend.

My wife will probably not admit it but I am fairly positive, her only real goal was to get through treatment so that she could go back to trying to have a baby. This, more than anything else was her mental issue with the breast cancer. Everything came back to that one thing. When we talked about surgical options, one of the reasons that we chose to try a second lumpectomy was that she wanted to be able to breast feed when we had kids. You really need to walk the line between being supportive of this issue and making sure that she is ready for the possibility that she will not be able to have kids. And if you are a guy with a biological clock ticking away, you need to come to the understanding within yourself as well.

If you do not have kids and it is a huge issue for you, talk about it with your wife. I can say now looking back that I wish we would have had kids earlier. It would have made all of the things that we have been through so much harder in many ways. But I think it also would have alleviated much of the emotional pain that my wife has gone through. Possibly some of the physical as well.

Here is another place where you need to have a conversation with your family and friends. We had a few friends that we were pretty close with that try to never bring their kids to see us because they think it will upset us. It does sometimes. But we also want to be a part of their kids lives and watch them grow up. So we had to tell them to stop leaving the kids at home and bring them over.

Then there are the folks that are just totally oblivious to how we might feel about it. They drone on and on complaining about their kids or how wonderful being pregnant is. We never want to have anyone not enjoy their pregnancy and baby because of us. But maybe folks should think about who they are talking to sometimes.

13 BABIES R US

It ends up back where you start. We were just starting to try to get pregnant when Jen was diagnosed and now after all was said and done.....we were back to trying to get Jen pregnant.

This has its' own set of ups and down and various mental and physical issues. Our oncologist was not what we are going to call highly in favor of us trying to have my wife carry a baby. She felt that having elevated estrogen levels for that long was just throwing fuel on a smoldering fire.

So the first thing that we did was think long and hard about what was important to us. This was a very sensitive topic for us to discuss. I had to find a way to convey to my wife that I loved her. That she was the most important thing in my life and that I did not want to risk her health for any reason. Then I had to at the same time convince her that I did want to have children with her but was also fine if we did not have children of our own. I was perfectly happy being cool Uncle Mike with a beach house and a boat. Not an easy thing to pull off. The last thing I wanted was for us to try to have kids, fail, and have it come back to me "not wanting it enough".

I will freely admit that I was very concerned about her ability to walk away from it if we could not have children. One of the few Lifetime movies I have ever watched was about a woman who went nuts when she could not have kids and the husband has to put her away. Given the irrational conversations I had been having with Jen about the subject, it was a huge fear of mine.

So after a couple of weeks of thought, we sat down to make a decision. For me, it was having my wife live a long and healthy life by my side. For my wife, it was to live a long and healthy life by my side…with children. So we decided to make a go at it.

There are lots of options out there from trying naturally to surrogacy to adoption to various drugs for having it yourself. We actually had a couple of people offer to be surrogates for us but neither of us really felt comfortable with that idea. We are both pro adoption but as a last resort. So we came up with a plan and ran it by our doctors.

Our plan was that we wanted to try naturally for 3 months and if that did not work, we would go straight to IVF (invitro-fertilization). We know that is not much but we felt like we should at least give the cosmic karma a shot at saying it was sorry for the last couple of years and here's your baby. Yeah, not so much.

So before we even got to the good trying to make a baby part, we had to find a

specialist to work with. When we had
first been diagnosed, we went and saw a
doctor in case we needed to freeze some
of Jen's eggs or something. He had told
us at the time that we should not worry
about it and most of the time, women had
viable eggs post chemo-therapy.

We tried to go back to see that guy but he
had moved his practice somewhere else.
So we saw another guy who was
recommended to us by several people
who had used him for fertility issues that
were not cancer related. He walked in to
the appointment having obviously never
looked at our file and had no idea who we
were or why we were there other than that
we needed help to have a baby. As we sat
there for 15 minutes while he read our
file, he finally looked up and said "I see
you have had cancer...you are going to
need to see a specialist. I cannot help
you". O.K., so the first thing out of my
mouth was "Aren't you a specialist?" His
response was a 5 minute lecture about
how he only took patients that he knew he
could get pregnant and that he had to keep
his statistics (90%+ pregnancy rate) high

and he felt we were 50-50 at best. In all of this, I had never come so close to pimpslapping a doctor as I did this guy. Are you serious????? Thankfully, Jen was fast on her feet and got us out of there prior to me saying anything further.

The next guy we went to see was at the hospital's Fertility Clinic. He was great. He had already looked at our chart, he was familiar with Jen's oncologist and offered to copy her on all of our records so that she was in the loop. He explained that there were certain drugs that he thought were a bad idea with Jen's history and we laid out a plan for the whole thing.

He had us run a bunch of tests to see if it was even possible. They determined that Jen had a decent supply of eggs that looked healthy and that some of her hormones were working at normal levels. But not all of them were functioning correctly. So we were going to need some low level drugs to help get her body

rolling in the right direction. I like to use
the analogy of a woman's body (as it
pertains to reproduction) as a hallway of
doors. Each door is locked. Each
hormone opens one door and then another
hormone opens that next one and so on.
But if one of the middle doors is closed,
the rest cannot be opened. Jen needed
some help opening a few of those doors.

Then I got to go take some tests. While
mine did not involve needles other than a
simple blood test, it is really not all that
cool to masturbate in a doctor's office.
First, the "collection room" (seriously that
is the nameplate on the door) is in a
hallway across from a bunch of offices.
So as I am in there mastering my domain,
I can hear them talking about where they
are going for lunch. Not sexy. Secondly,
they make you show ID and sign a bunch
of paperwork proving it is you before you
give them a sample. I mean, are people
sending in a stunt double? I have heard of
people using a fake ID to take someone's
drug test but this? I am normally an open
person when it comes to sex (if you have
read this far, you have figured that out)

but by this time, I felt dirty. Then they have a nice little couch and flat screen and a selection of porn for my viewing pleasure. Again, since I can hear the in depth discussion of the lunch menu at the local restaurants, I am sure they would be able to hear the "brown chicken..brown cow" music from "MILF Hunters 7". So I chose to forgo that part of the experience. On my test day, I went at lunch on a day I was working. I could not even look anyone in the eyes the rest of the day.

My tests came back with good news and bad news. I had some great little swimmers but there were not a lot of them. It looked like many years of contact sports had taken a toll on my testicles. So it looked like we might need to go to IVF. We decided to try out a couple of months anyway but no babies came out of it.

So we went back to the doctor and started looking at the IVF procedure. If you are not familiar with this, they basically take your sperm, her eggs, make an embryo in a Petri dish and then put them back into the woman. For me, it involves some further quality time with a cup in the "collection room". For Jen, it involved lots of drugs, daily injections and some radical hormone surges.

Our first step was to go to a seminar for couple looking to start IVF. This was I think the first day that I realized what we were about to do. It had all been sort of theoretical prior to that. We were by far the youngest people in the seminar and the only ones that were there because of cancer issues. So as they were showing the women the little tiny needle that would be used to inject themselves every day, the other women were lamenting about scars and pain. They made each woman give themselves an injection of saline just to see how it worked. The others struggled or complained. Jen just took it, jabbed it in and handed it back. My little hardass.

Once we met with the doctor and put an exact plan in place for when we would start, we had got a cost for the whole thing. And we started figuring out how to finance it.

Babies are expensive when they show up naturally. And since everyone knows how badly people want babies, everything having to do with getting one in this situation is incredibly expensive. And none of it is covered by insurance.

So we talked about what we wanted, how many times we would try this before we gave up, and how much we were willing to pay to do it. We decided that we would not empty our saving but would instead take out a loan for it. A hefty loan. Luckily, we had just paid off the last of her other medical bills, a car, and my student loans from college. What was going to be a slush fund was instead going to pay back the baby making loan.

As a man, one of the strongest
evolutionary forces that we contend with
is the desire to care for and support our
wives. Many men think this involves
working so hard that they make enough
for their wives to stay home and not work.
The culture and media reinforce that with
shows like Desperate Housewives. I have
many friends who think I am a bad person
for not wanting my wife to be able to stay
at home. But even I could not look into
my wife's eyes and say we could not do
this because of money. So we went
forward with it. She actually did well
when we talked about only doing it once
because of her health and so as not to
mortgage our entire lives for this.

We went forward with the plan and
started down the road to IVF.

Jen started on her course of drugs that
stimulated her ovaries into giving up the
goods. This involved daily injections for
a couple of weeks in her belly. But it
worked really well. When the time came,
they were able to collect 17 eggs. An

impressive number for a normal woman, let alone my wife with all that she had been through. I gave my portion of the chromosomes over and they were combined to make a stack of little embryos.

A couple of days later, we went back and they put two little us's back into Jen. We even got pictures of them in the petri dish prior to implantation. It was terrifying and wonderful all at the same time. Jen went home for bed rest for a few days and started the next set of injections (progesterone) in her butt for 10 weeks. Good times.

This happened to be over the Thanksgiving and Christmas season so lots of parties and dinners to go to when you have to give your wife a shot in the butt at pretty much the same exact time every night. I was waiting to get busted by the cops considering the number of times that it happened in a parking lot in the middle of the city. "No officer..it's not heroin…no…seriously I don't need to get a cavity search".

It was exciting but we were still nervous that it might not take. I would not let her dance other than slow songs at Christmas parties. No sex, no lifting, nada. And it worked. We went in and her blood tests were positive for a pregnancy. We were stoked to say the least. We kept going back for more blood tests every few days to make sure that things were progressing normally.

And then we had our first ultrasound. And we found out there were twins. Awesome. O.K., I really wanted to vomit because I was worried about having one, let alone two, but we were both incredibly happy. A quick note to any IVF doctors out there….you should really explain to the patients that there is still a possibility of the embryo's splitting after they have been implanted.   That's right folks, two could have become three or four. And not by spontaneous generation. Yes, I took a lot of biology courses, I know how twins happen. But at the time, it seemed like science fiction. As he zoomed by the 2nd little person inside my wife, he kept looking around with a very serious look on his face. My heart started to stop and I asked if everything was O.K. The nice doctor responded with "I am just checking for more". I politely explained that we only put in two and his response was "do you want me to tell you how many times I have delivered 2 sets of identical twins?" Again, doctors out there….that should be permanently filed under "Chapter One….Shit they should know in the beginning". Please move it from "Chapter 76…Things to talk about if it happens to come up".

So we came in hoping to see one healthy little baby and left with two. Kind of buy one get one free plan. Not exactly free all bills considered but it seemed like a bonus all the same.

At this point, Jen could not hold it in anymore and started telling anyone who she talked to.   It was still early but I understood and felt her excitement. After all that had happened, she wanted this badly and it was finally happening. I had told only a few people until I got a call from an old coworker who had heard from someone random. At that point, I knew the gossip was flying fast so I told people at my work. We even set up some special trips to see family and friends and tell them in person. Seeing the excitement on people's faces made Jen even happier. It had been a long time coming and I wanted her to be able to revel in it.

At this point we started several discussions at once. We talked about childcare, registering for stuff, and names. All three seem fun and cool. All much more complicated than that.

We started looking at childcare without any real idea of costs and differences. I will not go into much detail on this one other than to say what a huge racket this is. After weddings, childcare is the next biggest scam on earth. Seriously do 2

year olds need to learn foreign languages?
I have an idea that you should learn to
crap in a toilet before you learn to
conjugate French verbs.

The next adventure was registering for
stuff. Again...total scam. My lovely wife
had bought books that rated each thing
based on all sorts of different things like
safety, ease of use, user ratings, etc. I
showed up and was handed a laser tag
gun. No real idea what I was looking for
but ready to scan it when I found it. Jen
and I normally have somewhat similar
tastes in things. Granted much of the stuff
in our house I did not have an opinion on
but I tried to be really interested in this
trip. We started early, which for us was
like 12 pm. It happened to be NFL
playoffs that day so we negotiated being
home for kick off at like 6 pm.

We started with bottles for feeding the
little people. Given the double
mastectomy, there was no need for breast

pumps or anything of that sort. Guys, even though my wife knew this going in, it was still "a moment" for her that we needed to talk about and be bitter about for a little bit so try to not be blind-sided by that one. Then we started looking at different bottles and nipples and warmers and all of the other things that we did not have for 10 million years of evolution and still made it this far. My first question in this realm was this: Why are there different size and shaped nipples for every three months of age for like the first 2 years? I will freely admit that my nipples are wholly vestigial and that I have never breast fed a growing child. But I was unaware that a woman's nipples changed that much over the course of time. Wait.....oh you mean that they don't? That the nipple the kid gets on Day 1 is the same nipple he is sucking on Day 365? THEN WHY DID I HAVE TO REGISTER FOR 12 DIFFERENT NIPPLES??????? Oh right..because it's a scam. Seriously, I had women tell me about different sizes in the holes so that the kids got more faster as they got older. I say scam.

Then we moved quickly through the toys section which was the only one I was really all that keen on in the first place. Jen pretty much gave me the evil eye for about 2 minutes straight to make sure that I was not scanning anything. And it brought us to strollers. Now again, I did not realize that there were almost as many classes of strollers as there are classes of cars. There are the big ones with the baskets underneath and cupholders and IPod hookups. I refer to these as "BattleStrollers" because they look like little baby tanks going off to war. Then you have little yuppy jogging strollers for the trophy wives to run to the Whole Foods to get organic humus for little Creighton Ellington III's lunch. And the small strollers that people pretend they are going to use and not lug 40 pounds of crap around with them to go to the mall.

So in case you wanted to know, they do not make a lot of double strollers for 2 babies. They make them for someone with a 2 year old and a baby. Try finding one that holds 2 of the little carrier things. Now find one that is not hideous or big enough to roll a linebacker down the street. Yeah, so the stroller portion of the day's event was a bust.

Then we moved to bouncers and pack and plays and other things I am not what they are called. Again, these all seemed a little excessive. We kind of used a "how badly would this scare the dogs?" rule in looking at things. I did like the ones that let you hook up an IPod rather than just play nursery rhymes while rocking. My kids we going to be swinging to the smooth sounds of Eminem and Dr. Dre.

The cribs were next on the attack plan and it was tough to find one that we liked that we could configure two of in the nursery. Most of the ones that we liked were too big or one side was ornate and that limited how we could arrange the room. Oh yeah….and most of them were crappily built. But we found the ones that we wanted.

Now we went back to diapers and wipes
and formula…Oh My! I will admit that
by this point I was tired, hungry, and
overwhelmed. Plus these places are not
really built for people to move freely in.
You have little tiny aisles, plus people
that already have strollers and children,
plus big people (sorry pregnant ladies),
and then you are asking them to all pull
things down and try them out or stop and
stare at them to make a decision. I am not
what you call a "people person" and it
was making me cranky.

Anyway, I turned my back for 30 seconds
and Jen accosts some woman with twins
with 20 questions. Is this what we have
turned into? Talking with random
strangers in baby stores about what wipes
are the best? I couldn't do it. The one
thing during the pregnancy that bothered
me the most is that people somehow
thought that my wife being pregnant was
going to make me a nice person. That I
somehow wanted to stop and talk to them
about their kids or what daycare they used

and how to get rid of hemorrhoids. No dice. I was still the same asshole that doesn't want to hear about your issues. I was not looking forward to lots of talks with strangers about diapers.

Once I freed her from that nonsense, we were off into the magical world of things that go into and come out of babies. Much like the chocolate factory, it was a place of wonder and magic. And the site of our first "disagreement" of the day. Jennifer, armed with books, research, and opinions of strangers had very set ideas of which diapers, formula, and wipes were the best for our offspring. I, armed with a laser gun and approaching kickoff, did not care in the slightest what these were. I just wanted to scan them and get the hell out of Dodge. About 5 minutes into the "to warm the wipes or not to warm the wipes" thesis, I snapped. I politely (I thought) requested that she just tell me which one to scan and skip the lecture portion. This led to hurt feelings and me being told that I needed to be involved in the decision making.

We decided that we were done for the day. We would try again at a later time to finish up anything we missed.

Which brings us to names. Naming a child is possibly one of the most important things you can do as a parent, after staying off the crack during pregnancy. And, well, most of the time…just stay off the crack in general. But back to naming. If you give them a bad name, it can scar them for life. Remember the Hooker twins? Sheeza and Imma? Or Harrold Dick. Don't be those parents. And don't name your kid Apple or Blueberry. Life as a 7 year old is hard enough. Why make it worse?

So we started with a couple of books of every name ever written on a birth certificate. I went through and came up with a list of about 25-30 names for each sex. I gave it to my loving wife. She handed it back to me with the phrase "You have got to be shitting me". And

followed that up with "You know that
your children are going to be white,
right?". Each name had a different issue
for her. Some were too ethnic, some were
too weird and some, such as Darwin,
could not be used in the South with the
bible thumpers we deal with everyday.
Now, being well educated and well read, I
did like several names from mythology
and various literary works. My wife, who
is well educated but reads science journals
instead of Oscar Wilde, did not find these
names acceptable. Her list was very short
but she felt strongly about them. So did I
but not the way she wanted me to. We
were able to come down to 2 girl's names
that we liked and 0 boy's names that we
agreed on.

So we found out a couple of weeks later
that it was going to be a boy and a girl.
We were ecstatic. One of each and we
could be done and have the perfect little
family. We had the tests done for birth
defects and they came back clean. We
started planning showers and buying
cribs, and we were absolutely on Cloud 9.

And then my wife was admitted into the hospital.

14 ALL HELL BREAKS LOOSE

She had flown out to see her best friend
and go shopping for maternity clothes and
do girl stuff. I was home cleaning out the
attic to make room for all of the stuff that
needed to be cleared out of the nursery
and bringing down all of the things that
had been accumulating in the attic for
years for our future offspring.

She had been having some back pain and
generally not feeling all that well on and
off for a couple of weeks. We asked the
doctor and were told that it was normal
for pregnancy and that it should start to go
away soon. She started feeling worse in
Ohio and when she turned an orange color
and started to vomit, they took her to the
emergency room.

This was on a Sunday night when she was
supposed to fly back that night. They
admitted her and gave her fluids. They
started to run tests and saw that her liver
was enlarged the next day. I flew out

immediately. Now, for those of you that have not done this, I strongly suggest that you avoid showing up at the airport with no ticket, and buying one 45 minutes before takeoff. Especially a one way ticket. Can you say special one on one time with Security? I just barely avoided the body cavity search.

By the time I got to the hospital, they had already decided that she was out of their league and arranged transport to the local major University Hospital. I rode behind the ambulance in Jen's best friend's car. We got her over to the new hospital and she was admitted into the OB Labor and Delivery Ward.

Jen was in a great deal of pain and was practically burnt orange in color, including her eyes. When she went to the bathroom, her pee was the color of Coke.

Have you ever seen an episode of House?

The medical drama on Fox? Yeah, we
lived one. In fact, I will be very very
surprised if this case does not make it on
to the show in the coming seasons. The
doctors checked everything she has.
Twice. She had urine cultures, blood
cultures, sonograms, ultrasounds, CT,
MRI, NBA, NFL, MLS, and NASCAR
scans. The best part was that being in the
OB wing, they do not run most of these
tests on pregnant women due to small
risks in birth defects and complications.
So each time, we got to fill out a special
consent form to authorize the test and then
they reminded Jen what she might be
doing to the babies. Really good for her
mental state. And because of the
pregnancy, we went for some tests and
then got sent back when the technician
refused to do it on a pregnant woman or
just figured it was a wrong order and sent
us back to the room. Then to get them
rescheduled, you go to the back of the
line. So it was very slow going in the first
week. Yeah, I said week.

We had teams of doctors come in pretty
much around the clock to ask her the

same set of questions about her case history. Occasionally a new set would get thrown in. Like the infectious disease folks that asked when she last had sushi, traveled abroad, been checked for fleas and ticks.

After several of the rounds of tests, I finally pulled the doctors aside and requested that I sign the consent forms and that they stop pointing out to Jen the possible side effects on the babies. I explained to them that we knew when we started to try to have kids that there was a possibility that something would go wrong and that we would do whatever we had to do to save Jen. If we could save everyone, that was my first choice, but Jen was the priority. I do not say that lightly. It broke my heart as much as hers to put the twins at risk but it had to be done to find out what was wrong with Jen and to try to save them all.

So the first thing that they figured out was

that her liver was huge. Her pain was coming from the liver being massively enlarged and then being compressed upwards by her uterus filled with the twins. The top of the liver was pushing up against her diaphragm which was making it hard for her to breathe. They could not figure out what exactly was wrong with it and then started a new round of tests aimed specifically at the liver. By her lab results, we also knew that her liver was struggling, her bilirubin counts were through the roof causing the yellow-orange color. The rest of her blood values for liver function were also off. So they had narrowed it down to an organ for now.

At this point, she was really having trouble breathing because of the pain. This was causing her blood oxygen levels to drop, making it dangerous for both her and the twins. The answer from the doctors was to dramatically up her pain meds. This would take away the pain and allow her to breathe more normally. This worked except that now she was largely incoherent much of the time. So about

this time, the decisions became mine as
far as her care and treatment. Not really a
goodtime. She was still aware for small
bits and we tried to time her drugs around
when the doctors would be there so that
she could be as lucid as possible for test
results and the next round of decisions.

To deal with the problems of having tests
not getting done, they transferred her out
of OB to the medical step down unit,
basically just below intensive care. OB,
as wonderful as the staff there was to both
of us, was just not used to dealing with
this kind of case. Plus, they are normally
a happy place and we really were ripping
their hearts out with what was happening
with Jen. I truly felt for them. They
pushed very hard for her to get the best
care possible.

So we finally got to the point by Thursday
that she needed either an extensive MRI
followed by a small guided biopsy or just
a small guided biopsy. The doctors

wanted to do the MRI first to see the whole liver to get the best spot they could to take a biopsy. By this point, we knew that the 2 most likely suspects were cancer and what is called fatty liver disease. We said no to the MRI and asked that they go straight to the biopsy. We felt that they had to do that anyway and there were plenty of spots seen on the other scans to give them a really good idea of where to take the biopsies from. We needed to get an answer as fast as we could and start whatever treatment needed to be given. Jen was going downhill fast and we were starting to get concerned about the speed at which things were happening. They finally agreed and we sent her down for the biopsy.

The wait for the biopsy to come back was long. Not in actual time, we had preliminary results the next day. But in terms of the timeline of my heart and soul, it was fucking forever.

The doctors were stumped by her case since each thing that they thought it might be, had a symptom that did not match. Even the final two candidates seemed unlikely. The fatty liver disease normally does not present until the 3rd trimester of pregnancy, even in women with twins. And her small initial tumor, breast with lymph node negative status made cancer unlikely as well.

Guess which one it was.......the breast cancer was back. They were able to determine that it was the same breast cancer that she had before. So after all of the things we did, something slipped by. And it was throughout her liver and was very aggressive. They also found a small spot on the bone of her sternum and spine. They were not all that concerned with either of those spots since the liver was being ravaged. They decided to start chemotherapy that day with two drugs, Herceptin and Taxol. These were both IV drugs. And they ordered a third drug, Lapatinib, that was a brand new pill at the time. Now, a lot was happening and I was dealing with Jen and doctors and it slipped by me that they did not have the Lapatinib on site and someone gave her best friend the prescription for it and sent her to Kroger. I sort of heard it out of the corner of my hearing but figured I must have heard something wrong. They are not going to have this at a grocery store if they do not have it at a major medical center. So she came back a little later with empty hands. They ended up having to order it and the "rush order" took about 5 days to get.

So the next issue was that she was deteriorating quickly in all systems. They wanted to get her up to the ICU to get more attention and to start her chemotherapy. They had a bed ready in ICU but there happened to be a snow storm dropping all sorts of snow and ice on the city that evening. And it was shift change time. So nurses were unable to make it in, this included the oncology nurses who had to give her the chemotherapy. So Jen's nurse came back and apologized and told us that the chemo could not start until tomorrow because of the lack of staff.

Now, at this point we had been there for 5 days (6 for Jen) and I had slept little to none most of those nights. What sleep or rest I had involved me on the floor in the corner of a hospital room or at best on a hospital recliner that is not built for the Big Bone people like myself. In addition, I had been caring for my wife night and day and making literally life and death decisions.

I will freely admit that I came very close to losing it right then and there. I felt the blood start pumping through my veins and the adrenalin start to course into my system. You know how they say that someone can lift a car to get it off of a loved one in a life and death situation? I was about to lift that car and drop it on someone. But I caught myself. Barely.

About 5 seconds before I reached critical mass, I caught myself and forced a calm. I was probably still not polite nor nice about it but I did not grab anyone or scream (really loud) at anyone. As nicely as I could, I explained that every hour at this point was critical in saving my wife and unborn children. That 12 hours delayed was unacceptable. I asked who I needed to call or if I needed to go sit and watch a patient so that a nurse could come and administer the chemotherapy. I demanded that it be given that night. Thanks to the nurse on duty at the time, we were able to make it happen. She called directly to the top nurse on duty and explained the situation. They were able to shift staff to make it happen. We are deeply in debt to that nurse. I am pretty positive that those 12 hours made a difference in my wife being able to walk out of the hospital months later.

By this time, Jen's mother had flown into town and had a room at the local hotel. She was definitely struggling with her daughter being so sick. I tried to give her time with Jen and allow her to mother her some when possible.

One of the good things that was

happening during the hospital stay was that the staff was speaking with us in medical terms and not dumbing it down at all. This allowed us to get much more accurate results and discuss things with the doctors at a much faster rate and to make better decisions. This was definitely hard on some of the family at points. They struggled to keep up with the conversations and decisions as they happened on occasion. So I had to break out all of my analogies to explain things that were going on. I had been calling and keeping my parents, Jen's brothers and father up to date as well as a few other friends.

One of the hardest things to do is to keep having that same conversation over and over again. To keep telling people how truly bad off she was and that it did not look good for her or the twins. To continuously hear other peoples grief made it even more difficult for me to keep it together. I finally just kind of stopped calling people. I called her brothers and asked them to make a lot of calls for me. I just could not keep doing it and keep my own shit together. In a couple of days time, all of our family was there at the hospital so it made it easier to get info out.

The next issue that we had was that Jen's kidney's started to fail. She was having what is called Tumor Lysis Syndrome. Basically, the tumor was responding so well to the treatment that it was overwhelming her kidney's ability to filter the byproducts out of the blood and get rid of them. So she had to be put on dialysis. This was tough to see but she was swelling up to the point that her head was bigger than Barry Bonds. Her legs and whole body were stretched to the point that she was bruising and breaking blood vessels all over her body. This, combined with her increasing delirium was making me really think about things like quality of life and what she would want to have done.

They were pumping in drugs and pulling

out fluid so quickly that combined with
the dialysis, it started to play with her
blood pressure but they were able to
stabilize her pretty well. They had her on
continuous dialysis to both take out toxins
and also to take off the fluid that was
building up in her and causing the
swelling. It was working but they were
unsure of the amount of real kidney
damage that had been done and was
occurring. We would not know that for
months to come.

At this time, the delirium was increasing
almost hourly. The ammonia build up in
her body was very high. She was losing it
fast and all of her systems were going
downhill. It was at this point that I called
her brothers, father, and my parents and
told them all to come to the hospital. I
told them the truth that I did know if she
was going to make it more than a few
days and that if they wanted to come and
see her to please do so. I felt that it may
be time that they needed to come and say
goodbye. As much as I was planning to

continue the fight, I knew that it was going to be a close call at best and I did not want anyone to have any regrets about seeing her, even in that state, one last time. At this point, when she was awake, I tried to start having conversations with her about decisions that may need to be made and what she wanted. I tried to have the end of life discussion with her and she wanted nothing to do with it. She told me it would be fine and that she refused to consider that this could be the Endgame. So I was on my own if it came to making any decisions.

She continued to go downhill over the next few days. At about 4:30 am on Sunday morning, she called out to me to wake up because she thought she had wet the bed. She had not wet the bed. The twins had spontaneously aborted. I lifted up the covers and they were both there. Two perfectly formed 17 week little babies. There are some things that you see that haunt you for the rest of your life. That is one thing I will never be able to unsee no matter how long I live.

Thankfully, Jen was having a very lucid
span at that time. She was awake and
aware of the whole thing. I told her what
had happened and we called the nurse.
The nurse called for OB and they came
right up. Jen and I decided that we
wanted to hold them until their hearts
stopped beating. She held them for a little
bit and then gave them to me. We did not
want them to have their few moments on
this earth to be alone somewhere. I held
them and apologized for what had
happened. I did my best to explain that
we tried everything that we could to save
them too but that we had to try to save
their mother. I sang to them and cried.
Cried so hard I could not breathe.

OB took footprints and fingerprints of
both of them. They wrapped them up in
blankets and took pictures of Jen holding
them. I really cannot describe the
emotions that I went through that night. I
will carry the pain of that experience with
me for life. And I will carry the guilt for
not giving them a better life and doing

what I had to do to save Jen, even at the cost of their lives. At the same time, and I have even deeper guilt for this, I was relieved that the estrogen they were providing was no longer in Jen, and that we would no longer have to worry about if we were hurting them in our decisions.

We got Jen cleaned up and she got a nap while I handled telling the rest of the family that was there at the hospital what had happened overnight. Again, telling everyone else was extremely difficult. How do you tell people something like that? Even Hallmark does not make a "sorry your twins aborted and your wife might not live through the week" card. Even puppies and kittens could not make that card better. They brought the twins back up later that day so that Jen and I could see them one last time with the rest of the family, Jen was somewhat lucid for this and very matter of fact about it. She said that she felt that they sacrificed themselves so that she could live. She very calmly handled them and talked about how much they weighed and how long they were. She said goodbye to them and I sent them back down to OB. Later, we would have them brought back up again so that my parents and Jen's father who had just arrived could also meet them and say goodbye.

I was very happy that this happened when Jen was awake and aware enough to process it. Had it happened a day later, it would have been even harder. Unfortunately, this was the last time that she was lucid. By the end of the day, she could not answer the list of questions that the doctors asked each morning. What is your name? Where are you at? What year is it? Who is the president? What is your birthday? She got her name right and that was it. At one point, she kept trying to eat her oxygen sensor on her finger. Every time I would let go of her hand, she would look at me and try to eat it. It was like a zombie movie.

The next morning, her chest X-ray showed fluid on her lungs. The doctors wanted to put her on a ventilator to breathe for her. This was a tough call to make. So at this junction, she was out of it and I was the one making all of the decisions on her healthcare.

My choices were as follows:

Put my wife on a ventilator and hope that she could recover from liver failure, kidney failure, and fluid on the lungs. Oh and cancer. If she could not recover, I could have her taken off of life support later.

Let my wife die. I was assured that it would be a fairly quick and painless death. With the bilirubin and ammonia counts as high as they were at the time, they could not be sure that she would not have brain damage and they could not guarantee that she would ever come off of the ventilator.

Let's make that decision on sleep deprivation, drained emotions, and with

12 other family members having their own opinions. I decided rather easily to go ahead and do it. They intubated her and put in a nasal feeding tube as well. She had not really eaten in over a week and badly needed some nutrients. There were others that felt that it was a bad idea and that she should be allowed to die with dignity. I was told I was being selfish and trying to keep her alive for me and not for her.

It was right about this time that the medication that they had been giving her to try to get her intestines moving and bowels working kicked in. She went from no bowel movement for over a week to almost nonstop. So now she was hooked up to a dialysis machine and a ventilator, and shitting herself in the bed. I made sure that each time it happened, it was cleaned up quickly. And I helped each time to make sure that she was clean and comfortable. I asked them to put a catheter in so that she was not suffering that further indignity and so that she had to be jostled less for cleaning.

Also, few things piss Jen off like having anything on her face. So even sedated, she kept trying to pull out her ventilator tube. So she had to be restrained. So let's add strapped to the bed to her situation. That is something that was maybe even harder. When I or someone else was able to sit and hold her hand, we took off the restraint. But when we could not, it had to stay on for her own good. But it is extremely difficult to see your wife strapped down like that.

I was pretty much overwhelmed by this point. All of our immediate family was there, and it really felt like we were all there to say goodbye to her. One of her brothers had come for the weekend and then flown home. He got halfway there when we called and had him turn back around. She was about as critical as it gets. It was at this point that the head doctor for the ICU called me into his office for a private chat. He had several things to say. The first was that we had to return to normal visiting hours. People had basically just been rolling in and out as they pleased and having 3 or 4 in the room at a time. Some of them were getting in the way of the nurses caring for Jen and not even moving when asked to do so. He said that I was allowed to be there anytime I wanted since I was useful and not interfering with the nurses. Next, he told me that other people needed to stop pulling doctor's aside and asking random questions in the middle of the ICU. He had told all staff to deal with me and only me. I agreed with that part immensely. And finally he told me that he understood that I was seriously considering letting Jen go peacefully. He asked me not to do that. He had spoken with the doctors at his hospital and that he was not sure how much more they could do for Jen. But he knew that her oncologist at home was one of the best and that she might be able to do more. He asked that we have a conference call with her oncologist to see what she thought about it. I agreed to have that call and to not make any decisions until then.

Then I went out and gathered the group together and laid down the law as politely as I could. Of course, the people who were the ones being talked about did not agree and felt that it was unfair. But I stood my ground. I was not going to lose my ability to stay with her each night because of someone else.

During that week I did a lot of talking specifically with Jen's brothers. We have talked before about how close I am with them. I asked them to do a lot for me during that time. From making calls to talking to my work, to keeping me sane. They gave me their opinions when I asked for them and served as a sounding board for me when I just needed to throw out some ideas. I talked to them about the meeting and they suggested that I allow Jen's parents to sit in so that they had a better understanding of what the doctors said. I agreed to make that happen.

We had the meeting and during it, the

ICU doctor explained that Jen was stable enough to travel back to her home hospital if the oncologist from there felt that it was worth it to do so. She very much did. She felt that if Jen could be stabilized and transported, that she could devise a treatment plan to get her a quality life. She was willing to be much more aggressive than the hospital where Jen was at the time and was much more up to date on the cutting edge of research to try different things. She did not promise miracles or a 15 year life span. She said that once she was there and stable, they could better evaluate Jen and treat her. She told us that the median lifespan for her diagnosis of metastatic breast cancer was 4 years. I would take four years, no questions asked. I thanked both doctors and told them that I would think about it and get back to them in a couple of hours.

I again gathered up the family in a consultation room and told them about the meeting. I explained to them that it was not a democratic vote and that I would be making the final decision based on what I felt was best. But that I wanted to hear their input and thoughts on it. Most felt that it was a good idea to get her to her home hospital and oncologist and to give her a chance to beat the cancer for at least a few years if not more. I left the room and went in to talk to Jen about it. I know that she could not answer me but I needed to talk to her because I talk to her about every decision I make in life. I thought long and hard about it and decided that she would want every chance to fight this. That she would want me to keep fighting out here so that she could keep fighting the cancer inside. I decided to give her whatever systemic support that was needed to keep her alive until her cancer could be knocked back enough for her to make a comeback. I told her doctors to get her to back to her home hospital as soon as they could do so.

I truly hope that none of you ever has to make any of these types of decisions. It is difficult to really fathom the woman that you love not being there. And being the one that has to make the choices that lead to her living or dying is one that is hard to think about even in the abstract. I had to decide what I really thought that the outcome could be. Could she walk out of the hospital for a substantial time someday? What amount of time would I consider substantial? Would she approve of what I had done? Or would she wish I had let her go peacefully to be with the twins wherever they are? How long would I let it go before I decided it was over? What was considered progress in this situation? If her liver function got better but the fluid on her lungs got worse, what would I do?

A million questions and scenarios went through my head in those days. Some were just soul sucking pain that was not really actual thoughts as it was the total absence of all love and happiness in my body. Sometimes I could not breathe and was racked with sobs that I could not stop. Some were strange such as how would I stay in the house and live the lifestyle that we live on a single income? Could I pay the bills each month by myself?

Some had to do with how I could possibly
move forward with my life. How would I
explain this to our dogs? This may seem
stupid to some of you but I was really
concerned about this. They had not seen
her in weeks. She had left for a visit and
just never come home. I had a dream one
night that I paid extra to be able to bring
them into the funeral home to say
goodbye to her. I thought that if they
could see and sniff her body, that they
could better understand. I will be honest
and say that as hard as all of this was, I
may have had the worst breakdown when
I did eventually spend a night in my own
house. And Kobe and Brooke kept
looking for Jen. Running to the door like
I had left her in the car or something.
They did not know what was going on.
Did not understand that Mommy was very
sick and may never come to see them
again.

Once I had made the decision to go, they
put the ball in motion. She was accepted
as a patient in both the oncology and ICU
at home but they had no beds available. I
was told that as soon as a bed was open,

we were going. And at 3 am a day later, I was woken up and told that a plane was on its way. I got up, gathered all of our accumulated stuff, and made the cold ass walk through downtown to the hotel. There I showered and put a bag of essentials together for the trip and gave the rest to my parents to bring back with them. They happen to live about an hour away from us. Then I hurried back to the hospital making calls as I went so that the others could come and say goodbyes before we left for home.

And then we got word that the plane was having mechanical issues and had turned around. But that they were trying to find another one. And at about 3pm that day, the ambulance arrived to take us to the airport. Jen was strapped to a stretcher and all of her lines were hooked up to portable pumps and off we went. This actually took quite a bit of time and effort as she was full of lines and was getting many drugs and fluids simultaneously. We eventually got into the ambulance and took a fast ride (lights and sirens going) through the city to a local executive airport. I am not sure what model jet we were on but it was tiny. Two pilots up front. Jen on her stretcher along one side, the medical staff of two at her feet and hips, and me at her head with my feet against the back of the pilots chairs. The inside was rigged out like an ambulance with all of the things needed to transport the sick and injured. This thing moved though. We never got up very high once we took off. They fly under commercial traffic and have the right of way so they pretty much just go straight to the destination full tilt. From take off to landing was under an hour for what takes an 8 hour drive. Then back onto another ambulance to race to the hospital. We went in through the basement and straight up to the ICU. And as I took my second step in the ICU, I was soundly told to leave.

So after flying her in here to a hospital that I had never set foot into (we had always been in the cancer clinics), with a wife in critical condition, I was in a

waiting room that was filthy, with the
dregs of humanity. By this point, I was a
physical and emotional trainwreck. I
could barely walk upright because of my
back and I was pretty much crying every
five minutes. And then comes a nice
nurse to pull me into a conference room
and lay down the law that things were
different at this hospital. She told me that
she understood that I was allowed to be
with Jen nonstop at the previous hospital
and that it was not going to happen here.
That they would let me see her quickly
that night after she was settled in and that
I would then be made to leave. No
exceptions. I was told that they would
call if they needed me. That pretty much
put me over the edge. I curled up into a
little ball in the hallway and cried like it
was my JOB. On top of that, I did not
know where I was. All of Jen's
treatments and appointments and all of
my work things were in the clinic building
not the main hospital. I had no car there.
In fact, I did not even have any cars at
home. One was at a bar in the city and
one at my office. I did not know how to
get out of the hospital nor where to tell

someone to pick me up.

I eventually got to see Jen for a few
minutes and saw her settled in for the
night. I answered stacks of questions for
the doctors and nurses about her case, her
allergies, when various lines and ports had
been put in, etc. And then I was bid
farewell. I called a friend and she came to
pick me up. She was just as unfamiliar
with the hospital as I was so it made it
interesting to find each other. Going
home that night was difficult for many
reasons.

15 HOSPITAL NUMBER 3

Jen settled in to the new ICU and started to get a little better each day. I was still hanging on by a thread but starting to feel some hope for the first time in weeks. We started off by redoing every test that had been performed in the other hospital over again at the new one and taking out every port and line that came with her and poking more holes in her so that they all matched up with what this hospital wanted to have done. For any hospital administrators that stumble across this book, I would appreciate it if you could talk to the folks in your hospital and see if you could make sure that this does not happen when you get transfer patients. If it needs to happen because something is infected, go ahead and do it. But just so that you can say that you did it, well that is just arrogant bullshit. It's like no cellphones on airplanes, everyone knows its bullshit nowadays but we have to follow it. Anyway, it just gave her more holes and less options for them to put IV's in down the line because they had pulled out perfectly working IVs and could not get back into those veins later. But I digress.

It was also during this point when Jen had the only nurse that I did not like during the many weeks of her incarceration. After being as helpful as possible at the previous hospital, being allowed to participate in my wife's care, and being present for all but the highly invasive procedures, this particular nurse made me leave the room every time she went near Jen. And then it was an hour before I could get back in. Over the course of 12 hours, I was in the room for maybe 5 of them. And when I asked to see a doctor because all sorts of things were being done to Jen without me being advise or consulted, she refused to even bother calling a doctor. Then I complained about being kicked out of the room for Jen to get a blood pressure check and she told me I had been in there all day and that she did not know what I was talking about. I felt bad for a few days because I went off on her in the hallway. But then much later in this saga, I saw her on duty and went to apologize and got pretty much the cold shoulder, so I felt more like it was not me as much as her lack of people skills.

The biggest thing helping Jen at this point was her feeding tube. She had not eaten much in the past weeks and was badly in need of nutrients. So the feeding tube was shotgunning her as much goodness as her stomach would take each day. And she got dramatically healthier during that time. To the point that they had to keep upping her sedation to keep her under and calm. And finally one morning, the chest X-Ray came back clean and they decided to move forward with getting her off of the ventilator.

So they backed her sedation down for a day and then tried it first thing in the morning. They pulled totally off of sedation and she responded to some minor commands and they gave her the green light. I left the room so that they could pull everything out of her and when I came back, she was awake and spoke to me for the first time in over a week. Apparently, after pulling everything out, they tried to put a feeding tube up her nose to continue her nutrition. She fought them with everything she had left. Her first words to me were "don't let them put that thing back up my nose". I explained to her what was going on, that she was back in her home state, and that she was getting better slowly. Then she saw both her mother and father walk into the room together and asked me "did I die?", because they were seldom in a room together to say the least.

Jen progressed rather quickly from there back to relative health (in comparison to where she had been). She was drinking fluids and eating small amounts of jello and applesauce the first couple of days off of the ventilator and then was able to move to the Oncology unit and out of the ICU.

The Oncology ward was better because

she had a private room, a recliner, a bathroom, and I could stay there with her at night. She was still very weak and sick but getting better each day. At this point, I went back to spending basically every minute with her. I slept at the hospital in the recliner or on the floor (I eventually went out and bought a sleeping mat from REI that is made for putting under sleeping bags when you camp). I left for a bit every couple of days to go home and change clothes, see the dogs, go to the chiropractor to fix my back from sleeping in the hospital, pay bills, etc. I also went to the store and bought a laptop so that I could get some work done and also to allow her to watch movies and shows. But other than that, I was bedside. Jen could not mentally remember things that had happened to answer doctor's questions, remember what they said to tell me, or make decisions on her care when they had to be made. So I needed to be there to do those things.

I can't lie and pretend that this was not hard to do. The weight of pressure from these decisions, caring for her mentally and physically 24 hours a day, dealing with family and friends, and getting little sleep (and none of it comfortable) was wearing on me mentally and physically. About the second week at this hospital, I started to really struggle. Physically, my back started to go and I could barely walk or bend over. I was losing weight from not eating, and just generally falling apart. Mentally, I was starting to lose it and my memory was getting hazy on things, I was losing track of the time of day and day of the week, and was struggling to hold it together emotionally. With the immediate crisis over, I was having to deal with the mental aftermath of the loss of the twins and the potential loss of my wife, and the long term loss of the life we had dreamed of just a short while ago.

Thankfully, a couple of my best friends came down that weekend with their wives to see us. I needed it pretty badly at that point. I was able to leave the girls with Jen and get out to walk around with the guys just to talk and be out for a bit. I even stayed at home one night and had a couple of beers and some hot wings with them. It was sorely needed mental health time. But at the same point, it was hard to be home without her and I felt guilty for being home with them.

Once she was in the Oncology ward and allowed to have visitors, it was an avalanche. There were people there all day every day. She was showered with cards, gifts, and new blankets. People handmade some awesome blankets and quilts for us. A bunch of Jen's friends from the rugby team came by one night to give her a quilt and other stuff and had the room packed to the point that the nurse kicked them out to be able to get to Jen to change an IV. But it was good for us to feel the love and see people. Best of all, I arranged for her to be able to go to the lobby and had the dogs brought over to see her. I think that they thought they were going somewhere more exciting but they were very happy to see Jen and the feeling was mutual. We got to spend 30 minutes outside with our pooches. That was very healing by itself.

Things moved along from there and Jen
slowly got stronger from that point. She
was able to eat, with the help of tons of
anti-nausea meds. But finding things that
she would eat was a show. I basically
went down to the cafeteria or local mall
food court and bought one of everything
to bring back to her. Whatever she ate,
she ate. Then I ate the rest. Needless to
say, I stopped losing weight about that
time. But it was a constant battle to get
her to eat things. The nice thing with the
room was that it had a refrigerator in it to
store jello and things for her. She was
able to get out of bed and use the toilet
now so that we did not have to use the
bedpan anymore. That was a big day for
both of us.

She had some pretty nasty bed sores at
this point. The combination of swelling
and being in bed had caused her to lose a
lot of skin in the nether regions. So in
addition to helping out with various
wiping duties, I now was covering the
area several times a day in protective butt

cream. This is basically thick toothpaste that keeps it from getting worse and allows it to heal up. Fun stuff. This is not on my recommended activities list for a good time. But it has to be done.

So we trucked along with her slowly getting better and stronger. I was able to get out to work for a couple of hours at a time as well. The hospital had wireless so that I could work, update the Caring Bridge website, and get e-mail. Plus Jen and I could watch movies, TV on the internet, or shows from DVR that I had recorded to DVD. The time passed and one day many weeks later, we were told that she could go home.

We were excited and terrified at the same time. She was still very weak and on dialysis. I had no issues with being able to take care of her at home since I had been doing much of it in the hospital but she was very nervous. We finally went home on a Friday night. It had been a long day because of dialysis and because it seemed to take forever to get everything done to leave. When we finally left, it was too late to get some of the medications and some were going to take several days to get. Something it would have been good to know ahead of time. But we got home and it was pretty exciting for both of us.

For about 24 hours. Then Jen spiked a fever and started vomiting. We called the doctor and gave her some Tylenol. It helped but the fever kept spiking every 4 hours. By Sunday morning, we had decided to take her back to the hospital. Incredibly hard and defeating for us both. She was checked back in, and we went back to the Oncology ward.

They ran every test again and again and could not find any source of infection. They hit her with new rounds of antibiotics. Including the ones that caused her to be nauseous and have diarrhea before. In spite of no source for the infection and tons of antibiotics, she got sicker and weaker each day. One day during the every 4 hour check up, her blood pressure had tanked. I do not remember what it was but it was badly low (ballpark 50/20) and in came a pouring of doctors and nurses pulling everything out of the room and talking about calling a "Code Blue". Bad news. The good part was that Jen was fully conscious and aware and lucid. So she was obviously moving blood to her brain in spite of crap pressure. At this point they sent her back to the ICU.

The good news was that the nurses were much better and I was allowed to actually stay with her most of the time and at night. The bad news was that Jen's mental state was deteriorating quickly and she told me that she did not want any heroic efforts this time. No feeding tube, no ventilator, etc. I was starting to crumple myself with that news. She told all of her doctors and nurses the same thing. She told me that she was ready to die and could not keeping fighting anymore. As much as I tried to talk to her about this, she had made up her mind.

They continued to have no idea of what
the infection was but the doctors were
"Sure" that it was a couple of things that
involved minor procedures only to find
nothing. So they changed her antibiotics
to new ones, a couple of times.
Eventually she stabilized and she was able
to leave the ICU and go back to the
Oncology ward. During her ICU visit, her
brother's and sister-in-law were in town
for a couple of days. This let me get out a
little bit while they stayed with her for
times. Showers are good and under-rated
in general. You would be amazed at what
a little bit of sun and a hot shower will do
for your mental and physical well-being.

Back in Oncology, she again started to
turn the corner and get stronger and eat
more. At this point she had lost about 60
lbs. And the dialysis. Always a good
time. We had been there so long now that
we were on the third set of doctors that
had rotated through for some departments.
This resulted in us dealing with many of
the same communications issues that we
had worked out with other sets of doctors
previously.

Jen was also having a terrible skin reaction to some of the drugs. Again, no one was sure which one so they did a skin biopsy that told us nothing more than it was an allergic reaction. But she lost the top couple of layers of skin over her whole body. Legs, arms, stomach, butt, feet. Her whole body was peeling and itching. Her toe nails and finger nails were also starting to deform and eventually many fell off.

So in addition to being nauseas and in pain, she was also itching uncontrollably. Lots of fun. Also, they repeatedly put her on some antibiotics that caused her to have severe diarrhea. So at this point, I was lathering her up with various lotions and creams on a variety of body parts, and also waking up several times a night to help her back and forth the bathroom and clean herself up.

And then one day they told us to go home.

16 HOME SWEET HOME

After several weeks (47 days to be exact) and one failed attempt, we finally made it home for real. We were very nervous because of the first attempt but once we made it through the first couple of days, we started feeling better and better about it. The dogs were ecstatic. They did not leave Jen's side for about a week. Kobe lay under the recliner while she was sleeping and would return there after eating or peeing each time.

One of the best things we had during this time was that some friends of ours had set up a website to coordinate meals being brought to us each day. For about 2 months, we had someone bring us dinner every night. They were making dinners based on recipes from the kidney and dialysis website to help her kidneys. We called it "Operation Meatloaf" and then nobody brought us a single meatloaf. I eventually mentioned that we actually liked meatloaf and then we started getting them every night. We were getting extra meatloafs with other dinners so we put them in the freezer for later on. We also got a case of beer dropped shipped to us by one of my good friends and a box of steaks from another couple who lived in NJ and could not cook for us. I would like to take a second and truly thank each of the people who helped with this. It was very helpful to not have to cook while I was taking care of her and trying to do housework and job work and everything else. If you are ever in circumstances that require anything close to what we have been through (and I hope you are not) this would be something that you could ask someone to set up for you.

Another thing that was done for us that was incredible was that people set up a fund to help us and our family out with medical bills, airfare to the first hospital city, hotels and expenses there. They had donations sent to them and then they would send us cash overnight to pay for things. It raised many thousands of dollars and helped to offset the cost to our family to travel and be with us and also it enabled us to not worry as much about bills and missed work. We so deeply appreciated the help from everyone even though it was hard to accept charity and checks from friends and loved ones. It goes back to what I said earlier about people needing to help somehow. People were dumbstruck by what we were going through and they felt that they had to help in some way. For those of you that donated to the fund somehow, we were deeply touched that so many people cared for us. It allowed me to stay on FMLA for longer than I otherwise could and spend my time with Jen at the hospital. That is a gift that we can never repay.

We had to make some changes around the house like having a shower chair for her and she was still on dialysis so we had to accommodate that into our schedule as well. But we got by. Jen was eating better and was getting stronger bit by bit. After about a week, she was able to go up and down stairs but it wore her out to do so. So we tried to make sure that everything was in one place for her. She got strong enough after a couple of weeks or so for me to be able to leave for 3-4 hours at a time to go to the office. This helped her feel a little bit independent and it helped me to catch up a little but it was definitely hard to leave her there.

Also part of the fun was tracking all of her urine output. So I had an excel spreadsheet with her hour by hour pee output. And I would get home and she would have it sitting in the little pee holder waiting for me to count it.

I could easily go off on a tangent about how bad the conditions at outpatient dialysis clinics are but I will try hard not to do so. Let's just say that it is a crime against humanity. The whole process. We made several complaints including to the higher management and eventually got a meeting with the head nurse for the clinic. We pointed out that the aseptic technique was poor, that there was no doctor assigned to her case, and that she was feeling worse after treatment rather than better. Oh yeah, and she was told by a doctor (who did not even know her name) and several nurses that "Nobody ever gets off of Dialysis". That really helped the mental state for her. This was after every kidney doctor had told us that there was a good chance that her kidneys would recover at least moderate function. Jen finally got the attention of a nephrologist in the clinic who looked at her case. This is what we mean when we say take control of your own health care. He also did not think she would ever come off but he at least took a stack of blood and allowed her to do a urine study to see what was going on. At this point, she was making normal amounts of urine and had no more problems with swelling. But we were told that did not mean anything. Your body can make all kinds of urine without actually taking out the toxins like it is supposed to do. The urine study was us keeping all of her urine for 24 hours in a bottle in the fridge. Now I know that when you have kidney disease, it does not recover and that maybe that vast majority of people do not come back off of dialysis once they start. But as a medical professional, MAYBE you should be familiar with the medical case history of the person you are talking to when you say something. Maybe know their name at least. Honestly, had we left it up to anyone at that clinic to do anything, Jen would probably still be there.

Dialysis was also a very difficult schedule to keep up with. She had to go 3 days a week for 4-5 hours. It was on the opposite side of the city from work and everything else that we normally did. And she could not drive. So I would drive east to take her to the clinic with her getting more upset every mile for just having to go there. Then I would drive back across the city to work for a few hours and then drive back the other way to get her and take her home. She was pretty much always in tears and upset afterwards. Plus she just kept feeling worse each time even though she should have felt better. No one was allowed to accompany her during the hours of treatment because it was considered a "clean' area filled with blood filtering devices. The blood smell made Jen nauseas every time she went to treatment.

But we made the best of it. We packed up a bag with stuff for her to read or do while she was there. We filled her IPod with music so that she could try to rest and not hear the people around her, and snacks for while she was there. Since temporary dialysis ports are external and must not get wet, I ordered some port covers online that allowed her to shower regularly and we tried to make up a routine for those days.

After a few days, the urine and blood test results came back and they told us to not come to dialysis that day to see what happened. They wanted to let her body try having no dialysis and see if it kept up with removing the toxins and fluid like it was supposed to or not. If it was not working, we would know it based on her physical symptoms. The extra day became a week and then they re-did the blood and urine tests. And guess what? She did not go back to dialysis. So in case there are any dialysis clinic workers out there, try not to shit all over someone that tells you that they want to talk to a doctor. And if you are a doctor, make sure that you know the name and background of the person before you offer your advice. I realize from being through it that most of the folks in dialysis are poor, and many are not what I call well educated. But that should not allow the health professionals to treat them like my wife was treated during her dialysis experience. I know that AIDS and cancer gets most of the money but maybe someone could take a couple of minutes and look into making better equipment or curing the kidney diseases that cause people to end up that way. Just a thought.

We still monitor her kidneys, watch the salt intake, and check for swelling from time to time plus I chase her around with bottles of water every day. When she gets certain types of scans and other drugs, we take preventative measures to protect her kidneys as much as possible. We are hoping that portion of the battle is behind us for forever. Jen believes the dialysis was the worst of her treatments and the one thing that she will never do again.

17 GETTING BACK ON OUR FEET

 After everything that we had been through in the last few years, it looked like one of the hardest things to do was going to be simply just going on living our lives and rebuilding what we had left. The loss of the twins, the destruction of our plans and dreams that so recently had been coming true, was incredibly difficult to overcome on a daily basis. Years later, it still is.

We came home to a nursery that was more or less set up already. Toys were there. Cribs in boxes. Presents in cute little bags. We had decided in the hospital to come home and handle this stuff together. Jen did not want me to have to do it alone and she wanted some time to be in the there to start dealing with the loss. In addition to the stuff we already had, we kept getting things in the mail from the places we had registered and signed up for stuff. Want to make a bad

day worse? Get a box of free diapers or
formula in the mail. Or a letter
congratulating you on the birth of your
child. Jen just stopped getting the mail
for about 6 months. I would get these
things and just throw them away or take
things into work to people who had new
babies.

We received the cremated remains of the
twins and the pictures from the hospital
staff in the mail. I knew what it was but
had not opened it. It took us about 2
months but one weekend, we decided to
just do it. We went into the room and sat
down and went through all of the stuff.
We separated things into groups of what
could be saved just in case we decided to
do surrogacy down the line, what could be
donated or given to someone we knew,
what needed to just be thrown out.

We opened the box with the twins and
they were sealed in a beautiful little urn,
they sent us pictures and the blankets that
they had been wrapped in when they were
born. Jen had no real memory of any of it

so we talked our way through the whole night, the things that had happened, what had been said, etc. It took us the better part of the day to do this. It was one of the hardest things I have done but it did help a little to do it together and talk things through.

We also had to figure out how to move forward with our new lives. Jen was still on disability and we talked at length about if she wanted or needed to go back to work. We decided that her just sitting around the house was a bad idea and she went to talk to her boss about when she could come back and what she could do. It was decided that she would go back part-time (30 hours a week) as a slightly different position without some of the more stressful parts of her old job. She ended up going back part time in August.

She was getting stronger and even starting to go to the gym with me and walk on the treadmill. She was getting out more and

we were going out with friends and
starting to make our way back into the
mainstream of the world again. As
before, I had to be the person to maintain
the balance between pushing Jen to keep
moving forward and telling people that
"no" she was not ready for that or that we
could not make it someplace. We missed
some things that year, a friend's wedding,
a child's birthday party and some other
things because we either could not
emotionally handle it or Jen could not do
it physically. One of things that is not
talked about or thought of by most people
is the difficulty that those in our situation
have in social settings after such a
traumatic experience. Whether it is work
or a dinner party or a family reunion, it is
very hard to be constantly looked at with
pity. Most people do not even realize that
they are giving you the look. That "look
at her, I feel so bad for her" look. The
reaction from people and the attention is
nice in certain situations but it is hard to
see it day after day. Or you go to a party
and some person starts to talk about their
horrible kids and then either they realize
halfway into the conversation who they
are talking to and it gets awkward or they

have no idea who you are and what the history is and they just keep on talking and then ask if you have kids. When we say no, they start going on about how we should have them and we don't know what we are missing. Depending how we are fairing that day, it can put either of us over the edge. It is not something that goes away although it has gotten somewhat better with time. We try very hard to not shit on anyone else's good time. We love the children in our life, be they our nieces and nephews or our friends children. We dearly cherish our Aunt and Uncle status and spending time with all of them. But it does also hurt somedays. What help many days is our dogs (Kobe who has since crossed over the Rainbow Bridge, Brooke, and our newest addition Montana). They are pretty perfect, except for the shedding.

I never used to cry. I had exhausted my tears when my brother died and just few things affected me to the point of tears for many years. For a couple of days in February 2008, I cried almost nonstop. After that, I was able to tail it back to a few times a day. Now, as we move forward again, I am not nearly as indestructible as I once was. Maybe we just never noticed it before or maybe we just got hosed but it seems like every episode of every show that we watch is now about a woman with breast cancer or about babies or both. We had to turn off shows halfway in several times in the last couple of years. I can also assure you that these shows are incredibly inaccurate when it comes to reality. Even listening to the radio can be hard some days. There are a lot of songs about pain and loss. They did not used to bother me but now there are days even they can bring me to tears.

We have adjusted our schedules of both work and life to revolve around the treatment protocol that she is on. Basically, every few weeks she goes and gets IV treatments at the clinic. It takes from 3 hours to 6 hours depending on the day. The treatment is always the same, the time we spend waiting changes each trip. And then every 3 months, we spend a day where she gets scanned inside and out. Then we do not sleep that night as we wait until the next day to meet with the doctor to see how the scans look. If they are clean, or have no advancing cancer, then we keep doing what we are doing. If it looks like we are losing the battle, then we will switch to a new treatment. We have learned to just not plan anything that day or the couple of days afterwards when we can. I am able to schedule around work most of the time. We are both very lucky to work for companies that have been incredibly supportive throughout the entire process. They have allowed us to be flexible and work from home and laptop when needed. If I cannot go, we find someone else to keep her company that day. We have made friends that are on the same schedule that we see each time and have learned to find things to pass the time. We also chat among ourselves, read, or Jen answers questionnaires that I ask her the questions in silly accents to make her laugh while we do it.

There are still frustrations to be had. Every time we go for a round of scans, we argue with the radiologist about Jen getting the contrast agents. She is not supposed to get them because they could be toxic to her already damaged kidneys. But the radiologist does not get as good a picture without them. So they trot out each time and give us this look of condescension and tell us how they are right and just to do what they say. Then we explain that NO, we know what we are talking about and see, there it is right in her chart, NO contrast agents. Good times. I think we have had maybe one time that they have not delayed the scans so that they could talk to the oncologist to be "sure" that there should be no contrast. We do the contrast every 3rd scan as a compromise and Jen takes special pills and gets extra fluid as protection for her kidneys. And we hope for the best.

Sometimes we get the best and sometimes we do not. After almost 2 years of good scan results, they found 2 new spots on her liver. Neither was large and the blood work looked fine but it signaled that something was starting to change and that the cancer may be started to fight back. We were told not to worry about it yet, to keep the treatment going on schedule and then we would evaluate the scans in another 9 weeks to see if there was any further or new progression of the cancer. This happened to correspond to the Christmas holidays and we kept the news mainly to ourselves so as not to freak people out and make them worry. About 4 weeks shy of that next round of scans, Jen started getting headaches. They were minor and transient at first but started to get worse and more often. So we asked for her to get a brain MRI just to take a look at it. We tried not to jump at shadows and we really thought it was just stress or something. But she was due to go on a 7 day SCUBA cruise the following week and we did not want her to be out in the middle of the ocean and have a seizure or something.

Well we got the scan and the next morning, the Oncologist called and told

Jen the news. The cancer was in her
brain. In multiple spots. She had been at
work when she got the call and could not
drive so a co-worker brought her to my
office. I stopped what I was doing and we
just went home. Jen's oncologist had
already started everything in motion and
had arranged for us to see the top
specialist in brain radiation oncology at
the clinic. Any other time that she had
referred Jen to someone, it had always
been an "I am not even sure who it is but
the nurse can tell you" or "go see so and
so, but then come back and we will talk
about it". This time, she told us who to
see, that he was the best and to do
whatever he said to do. She also
personally called ahead and made sure
that we got fit in the next day and that he
knew all about Jen.

I want to take a second here and just talk
about how incredible Jen's oncologist is.
I cannot explain the relationship that we
have developed with her over the years.
She knows us the way that no other doctor
knows us, our life, our goals. And she has
let us into her life as well. She has
touched our lives and allowed us to touch

hers. For this we are very thankful because we know that we have someone on our side and that we trust to be honest with us, and care about Jen as more than just a patient ID number. Thank you.

So we saw the radiation oncologist the next morning. This was outside of our realm. Neither of us were really that knowledgeable about the radiation treatment side of things like we were on the chemotherapy side. It was a new part of the clinic we had never seen, a new regime that we had not been through, and as we were about to find out, a whole new set of issues and side effects.

We met with the radiation oncologist and he and his staff were very good about explaining what the process was and what to expect. Given how active and intelligent Jen was, they wanted to opt for a longer treatment plan using lower doses each time. So instead of 10 higher doses, she would get 20 lower doses. They put her on steroids to try to get the brain swelling down and to stop the headaches. Also, the brain was about to get pissed off at being irradiated so the steroids would help with that as well. Also, Jen would lose her hair again. No big problem there as she was pretty comfortable being bald at this point. She would get fitted that morning for her mask that lined up the radiation and held her head in place and then start treatment that afternoon.

The other issue was that because of the risk of seizures, Jen would not be able to drive during treatment and for quite awhile afterwards. Ouch. Jen was not happy at all about that one. Neither was I honestly because it makes it hard to get her around when she cannot drive and also when you have to have her to radiation 5 days a week for 4 weeks.

So we got her set up, treated and we went home from there. And of course there was a snow storm that night. I would like to consult a meteorologist to find out the link between cancer and snowfall. In each of the cases in which Jen's cancer has "flared up", it has snowed. There was a big snow storm when she had her first biopsy, when she went into the hospital the 2nd time, and now. This time was only about 4 inches but where we live, that literally shuts things down. As a reference point, it snowed Friday night to Saturday morning. Schools were out until the following Thursday. And they went in late that day. Now, we have a pair of Jeep 4x4's and we got up the next day and went to her appointment. We were the only ones there besides the staff that had stayed in a hotel the night before. Craziness.

So we arranged for people to take her back and forth to treatment most days so that I could still go to work. Unfortunately, the clinic and the house are on opposite sides of my office so it would have been hard to go home to get her and then go to treatment. It was definitely difficult to not be with her for the treatment each day but again, it lets others help and it was something that I really did not have to be there for each day. I still went on the days she saw a doctor or went for check-ups.

This was the first time in all of this that Jen could not drive for any length of time. Sure there had been times during surgery or treatment that she did not feel up to driving or driving for long or far away. But this was the first time that she was under orders not to drive for months. This was due to the possibility of seizures as a side effect of the whole brain radiation. They did not want to have her endanger herself or others behind the wheel when she could have a seizure and cross lanes, etc. This caused a whole new area of problems when it came to both getting her to where she needed to be and also in her sitting in a house by herself for long periods of time. The bulk of the day on most days.

The first issue was getting her around. Like I said above, her treatments were in the opposite direction from my office so it made it very difficult to go home and get her, then go to treatment, then go back home to drop her off, then back to work. So we settled on asking for a lot of help to get her to treatment each day or at least to get her to my office. Some days, I would just go in extremely early, then she would get a ride to me, and we would go from there. Other days, someone else took her then they went to lunch, etc., depending on how she felt that day. We again are very lucky to have family and friends that are willing to help out and were able to fill in whenever needed.

The staying home by herself part was much more tricky. When she was having days where she was tired and slept for 18 hours of the 24, she got by fine with a little internet access and 300 cable channels. However, once she was feeling better, she was dealing much more with depression (side effect of the brain radiation as well as side effect of finding out you have cancer in your brain). Getting her out of the house as much as possible became a necessity. Our friends again jumped in to the rescue and tried to coordinate picking her up for a day out as often as she felt up to it. We have a couple of friends with small children who are currently stay at home Moms that would come get her and go to the park or shopping, or just hang out for the day to give her company. Also, many of Jen's co-workers are on a 4 day work week with different days off (as she used to be before all of this started up) and would come by on their days off in the middle of the week to get her out. Something as simple as being able to go to the grocery store during the day was deeply helpful both to us as a couple and to her mental state of independence and being a useful member of society. She struggled with both of these aspects during this span.

She had good days and bad days. Only once did she have any major meltdown. She over did it one day and had a meltdown while out with someone else for the day. She was fine the next day but it was scary at the time. I also was not notified of the issue until I got home that night which was more than a little bit after the fact. While I understand the idea of "not bothering" me and that she was taken home and was resting when I got home, it is something that needs to go on the Instant Notification list for the husband.

We had this issue several times over the years where someone who was watching her at the time made the executive decision that I did not need to know something in a timely fashion. If you are ever in the position to be caring for someone that is sick like this, always err on the side of notifying the husband. Let him decide if it was important or not. It is hard enough for me to not be with her and at her side when I think she is fine and feeling well and being well cared for. It is much more stressful when I am not there and I cannot trust that if something happens, I will not be instantly and accurately notified of the issue. It is not being helpful to let me finish my day at work even if there is not anything I can do at the moment. All it does is make the coming days more stressful because I am worried about what could be happening at home without me being told about it.

She had constant issues with stomach
aches from both nausea and acid reflux.
She had essentially an upset stomach for
about 2 months straight. Not much fun
for her and we were not quite able to get it
under control. But she powered through
and some things did help. One was a
wedge pillow (looks like a wedge of pie)
under her pillow which helped her to
sleep at an angle that kept the acid from
getting up out of her stomach and into her
throat. The other was the meds for acid
reflux that seemed to help it some as well.
Eventually we were able to win the battle
and get her back on the uptick.

At this point, in response to the cancer
trying to fight back, it was decided by the
Oncologist to put Jen back on an
additional chemotherapy drug that she had
been on a few years earlier. She had been
on the drug in the hospital for a few
weeks in the last bout with cancer. It was
a new drug and one of the most effective
out there, but it caused Jen to have a

severe rash on her whole body. The Oncologist felt that the rash was because there were so many other things wrong with Jen at that time point and that this time, it would work better. Neither of us was particularly convinced of this but we felt it was worth trying it.

So we started it on a low dose after radiation treatment was over. And in about a week, the rash was back. Not as bad and not all over at first but enough to make Jen feel itchy and bad when she was finally starting to feel a little bit better. One of the issues with this drug is that it has to be taken on a totally empty stomach. We were told to make sure that she had not eaten in 2-3 hours and then take it. We were doing it at night late but apparently Jen's metabolism was slow and still held food in her stomach after 2-3 hours. So we switched the timing up to take the drugs in the morning. This helped after about a week and the rash largely went away with only minor spots and flare ups.

There were other minor side effects that we noticed such as light and sound sensitivity during treatment, some eye sight things that were transient, but for the most part she did well during those months.

Her brain has had several flare ups in the past 3 years. Each time, we have gone back and she has had some kind of treatment for it. Sometimes it has been additional radiation when the tumors were growing again. The problem is that you can only give the brain but so much radiation in a lifetime. We are lucky that so far she has tolerated it extremely well given the problem others we know of have had with much less radiation.

She has had a brain biopsy which was pretty scary at the time. Several times she has had brain swelling that have caused minor issues such as numbness and tingling in the arms or legs. And the most recent issue has been swelling in the brain due to physical changes in the brain due to radiation itself over the years. Scar tissue in the brain is more or less how it can be described. We were in Europe touring Italy and other countries for an awesome vacation that we had been planning for a year. While there she started to have trouble with her legs giving out. It only happened a few times but on one she fell and hurt her knee. It impacted what we were able to see and do, but not by a lot. But the stress of it was affecting both of us. We landed on a Sunday and she had a brain MRI that week. It showed massive swelling in her making it difficult to see if there was new tumor growth. They put her into the hospital for high doses of IV steroids in an attempt get the swelling down. By a week after we came home, she was in a wheelchair and had difficulty walking all but very short distances.

The steroids were unable to bring the swelling under control. We were presented with few options. One was a

Michael Streicker

drug used for other cancer treatments that
was shown to reduce brain swelling in a
few cases. We chose to try this treatment
realizing that there were not many other
things that we could try at this point. We
were again confronted with the possibility
that this might be something that we could
not stop. She had the treatment and then
1 week later, she had another brain MRI
to see if it had helped at all. The doctors
were honest with us that if it did not, they
were not sure of what to do next.

We received the results and thankfully,
the brain swelling was going down. The
drug was working. We are not sure how
long it will work or if the brain will
stabilize on its own. But after 6 months
of physical therapy, rest, and treatment,
Jen is finally back driving again (after
another 6 month hiatus) and even starting
to do yoga.

The casualty this time around was Jen's
career. While her company was again in
our corner and wanted her to return, she is
just not able to do so anymore. She went

in and cleaned out her things and said goodbye to everyone. It was very difficult for her to do so. And it was hard on both of us to have her lose that part of her life after fighting to go back so many times. She gets a lot of energy from others and not having that each day was not great for her.

Michael Streicker

18 MOVING FORWARD, ONE STEP AT A TIME

The hard part in our day to day lives is planning for the future. We know what the prognosis is. But we also know that advancements are being made all the time. Do we start hitting the Bucket List? Live like there is no tomorrow? Or do we look long-term and say "we are beating this son of a bitch" and plan for our retirement? We have personally chosen the middle road. We have always lived for today more than a lot of people. We travel, we do things we want to do now and worry about later tomorrow. And we continue to do so. But we have also looked down the line and planned for the future as well. We put away money for later, we plan for future trips years down the line, we talk about the things we want to do when we build our dream house.

The sex issues are still there, even worse in some cases because she had her ovaries removed so there is no estrogen coursing through anywhere. But we have learned to get by and have made progress in this area. I rarely get embarrassed but when we had a specialist come and talk to us in an open treatment room and used third person to talk about my penis, even I blushed. But this is the one area where I would say there have been great strides made because there are companies that make products focused on women with cancer and their husbands. If you have not already, you should check into these. There are some excellent products out there that can help you keep that part of your marriage up and running.

One of the things you have not seen mentioned in this book much is religion. When you go through the things that my wife and I have been through in the last several years, often the first thing (and second) people start to hit you with is their religious beliefs and how you should pray and whatever god you are aiming at will make it all better. You cannot imagine the looks on people faces when you tell them "No thanks". I am all for

each person believing in and doing
whatever they personally have to believe
and do to make it through each day, let
alone get through cancer. If that means a
religion in your case, have at it. It does
not mean that is mine. And we were often
the subject of visits from case workers
and social workers that we there to help,
well mostly there to see what religion we
were so that they could send the correct
chaplain. Again, folks were incredibly
surprised when we declined their offers.
People mean well and we appreciate that
they pray for us and put us on their prayer
lists at their various churches. But if you
are not a religious person, don't feel like
you have to be to get through this or that
you have to accommodate anyone else on
that subject.

During Jen's second occurrence of cancer,
we connected with a group called the
Pathfinders. They are basically
somewhere between a support group for
women (and their husbands and families)
with Stage Four Breast Cancer and a
Cancer Concierge that provides help with
anything from explaining side effects and

test results to finding you a good masseuse or therapist. The person we have been lucky enough to work with has done wonders for Jen and also some truly helpful things for me as well.

They base their system on "The Seven Pillars of Personal Recovery". The pillars are: Hope, Balance, Inner Strengths, Self Care, Support, Spirit, Life Review. I am not a touchy feely person, I don't burn incense, and I don't do yoga. If you have read this far in the book, all of these facts were totally surprising to you I am sure. But these pillars helped Jen a ton. Her pathfinder also taught her a lot of coping mechanisms such as visualization, breathing techniques to relax and focus when stressed, and other things. There are also support groups some of which even involve the husbands.

We have been working with them for several years now and Jen still scheduled appointments to see her pathfinder and

attends group sessions as well. Also, the
pathfinder knows our treatment schedule
and almost always stops by to see us at
some point in the day to catch up. She
checks to see how things are going in the
cancer side of our life and also on all
other aspects. There have been times
when she has had counseling sessions
with us to work through certain issues and
these have helped us deal with things
much better than maybe we could have
without a little bit of professional help.

Which brings us to the issue of anger.
Much of Jen's was anger at the world, at
the hand we had been dealt. There was
also anger at me for following her around
with jello or anger at the person in the car
in front of us for not going fast enough. It
took me off guard much of the time.
Especially after working all day, then
coming home to take care of her, to be
lashed out at by your wife is a tough thing
to just brush off. Sometimes I was able to
do so. And sometimes I was not and
yelled back. There are days that no matter
how hard I tried, I could do nothing right
in my wife's eyes. When all you are

trying to do is what is right, it hurts for it not to be recognized.

My wife and I are both strong willed, intelligent and independent people. Prior to cancer, we "disagreed" on things from time to time. Sometimes this was a passing disagreement and sometimes it was major and required many discussions prior to a treaty being signed. However, after the cancer came back and Jen almost died on me, we no longer fought. She would lash out and I would maybe say something back and walk off but we did not really argue in any sustained manner.

I did not want to lose an hour or night arguing with her since I knew that my time with her could be less than I had hoped for in the long run. But this started to affect our relationship and our individual stress levels. Finally one night, over something I can no longer remember, we blew up. We both argued with both barrels full and let loose with all of the things from the past year that had pissed us off. It was somewhat nasty on both of our parts.

And then we both realized that it had just all been welling up inside of us and just came pouring out all at once. So we went in the next time we had to go to treatment and talked with the pathfinder about it. Got some advice from her, heard that it was O.K. to disagree even when Jen had cancer. And it helped us to talk things out better moving forward.

The pathfinders also arranged a meeting with several husbands of women in the program. We met and talked about what we had gone through. It was only a couple of hours but it was great to be able to hear how other men had dealt with things, to be able to answer questions that they had and have some of mine answered by them. I found the meeting very valuable and hope we get to do so again in the future.

The good part of our life is that we have had the opportunity to do some incredible things that we would not have done

otherwise. We have traveled to some
dream destinations, Jen has learned to
kayak and SCUBA dive, and we have
seen more of our family and friends than
we used to.

There have also been three organizations
that we have been able to be a part of that
have been fantastic chances to both see
and do things we would not had the
opportunity to do if not for cancer but also
to give back to others and help out at the
same time.

The first is the Foundation for Biomedical
Research. This group approached us
about Jen filming a Public Service
Announcement about the role of animals
in biomedical research and how important
they were in finding treatments and cures
for diseases like breast cancer. They were
intrigued by Jen being a researcher herself
while battling the disease personally. We
said yes and they proceeded to film the 30
second spot and play it nationally on

Youtube and on TV. It ended up winning
4 Telly Awards that year. Telly Awards
are the commercial and PSA version of
Emmy or Grammy awards. They are
made by the same people and it was an
honor for something we were involved in
to win an award at that level.

After the PSA did so well, they asked us
to consider filming a 30 minute show
expanding on that theme. They wanted to
follow us around the treatment process
and show Jen at work and how drugs got
from the labs to the clinics. We thought
about this for a bit prior to saying yes.
We are both very proud of what we do but
there are lots of animal rights people out
there that are not O.K. with it and bomb
houses and labs, and all around terrorize
researchers. We felt that it was important
enough to get the truth out there to the
public that we wanted to be a part of that
process. Animal rights activists had been
allowed to spread lies for too long and we
wanted to help do our part to educate the
public on how labs really were and the
incredible importance of research to find
treatments and cures.

They followed us around the clinic for a few days and filmed us going to scans and doctor appointments and treatment. They also followed Jen around her lab and we were very happy with the final result. When they had it done, they told us that they (FBR) wanted to throw a Gala to debut it and also to show it on the local NBC affiliate the next night. It ended up being awesome. It was literally the week that Jen finished radiation so it was hard to balance everything but we had almost 200 people there from all parts of our life and also from the research community. Family and friends from across the country came in for the weekend. It was at an awesome venue and there was anything from showing the 30 minute video to speeches given by Jen and her Oncologist, to just chatting with friends over wine. Everyone was invited to play in a golf tournament fundraiser the next day and then we had close to 100 people at our house for an authentic Pig Roast. It was a great time and all of these events were crucial to help Jen get back on track after being down for a month.

The second thing is that Jen was accepted as a model for a wine bottle label. This winery puts out several different wines each year and the labels are pictures of Breast cancer survivors. She was picked with 5 others that year to fly out to California and spend a weekend taking glamorous photos and drinking wine. The wine she is pictured on is actually very good and we have hosted several wine tasting events that have ended up selling quite a lot of it with the money going to breast cancer research and survivor programs.

And the last thing was a group called First Descents. This is affectionately referred to as Cancer Camp in our house. It is a charity that offers young adult cancer survivors (all types of cancer, not just breast) the chance to go to beautiful destinations in the USA to rock climb, surf, or white water kayak. Jen learned about this group from another model at the wine photo weekend. She applied and was accepted to attend one of the kayaking camps. She spent a week in Montana having the time of her life. She was energized by the common bond that the campers had and also by the dedication of the staff and volunteers at the camp. She came home with new friendships that have become positive support for her.

Overall, we have done our best to make the most of what at times has been a shitty hand. We travel as much as we can to see family and friends. We spend a lot of time just going places and doing what we want to do. It is a hard balance that we have struck between living for today, which many folks have done in our situation, and planning for the future. We hope and live as if there will always be a new treatment that works and maybe one day a cure. But we know that the worst is always possible as well.

As a husband, that may be one of the hardest deals to make inside. I do not like to say no to anything that she wants to do. Except Skydiving. Not going to happen. It may not make the best financial sense or be the wisest thing for the long term, but if we can swing it, I try to make it happen for her. But you cannot live indefinitely as if your wife will be gone in 6 months. Personally I have been told she had 12 hours to live and that was over 5 years ago. And I fight everyday to make it 60 more years with her. But you cannot just go on living as if you can take that trip when you retire either. You have to find a middle ground somewhere. And it can be very difficult to do so. Most of the time, either someone gets sick and they get better in a relatively short period of time or they get sick and die in a relatively short period of time. Either you fight it for a year and get better or your fight it for a year and lose the battle. But with the advances in medicine (through research by the way) that have been made, that battle has become a much longer one in a lot of cases. Which is wonderful because every extra day and extra year is worth the price.

But it can also wear you out. Every day, week month and year that you get to spend with your wife is wonderful. However, the constant stress of the medical ups and downs, going through treatments, and all of the other ailments that each new things brings, will take a toll on you mentally, emotionally, and physically.

Others get to pop in and out of your life and help out on occasion. They may come for a weekend or a week. But they still get to go back to their own lives. This is your life. It can be hard and it can wear you down. You have to really work hard to not let it do so. You have to work hard to keep your strength up so that you can keep going and can keep her going as well. I have been asked many times how I can leave my wife at home and go play sports or go to Las Vegas for a guy's weekend. My answer is that it keeps me sane. It is what I would be doing if my wife did not have cancer. It is what I enjoy and it relaxes me so that I can come back with my batteries charged to do what I have to do at home. Just as she goes to cancer camp, I go to Las Vegas camp. Or whatever it is that you do to relax. Fish, golf, camp. I don't care, just do it. Does that mean that I do not miss her? No, I do and it can be hard to be away from her much more than it was before all of this. But sometimes you have to have a little self-care of your own. Jen does the same, she travels with others and takes trips without me. I am not overly fond of this because I am extremely protective of her and worry about her when I am not around. But she needs a break from me as well. We try hard to mix it all together, her time, my time, and our time. Just as both of you are there for the hard stuff, you should both be there for the fun stuff.

We also try our best to give back what we can. Whereas we have always been the type to donate or volunteer time to a charity, we have found the need to do more when we can because so many people have helped us. We have seen so many people that do not have the support groups, money, flexible jobs, or marriage

that we have had access to over the years.
We have tried to think of ways that we
can help them. Some of it is giving
someone a Cancer Sucks button or hat,
organizing a team for a charity race, or
writing this book. We have really tried to
look at what we have been through as
something that could possibly benefit
someone else someday through our pain
and experiences. If any of this
information can help another husband or
couple, I will consider it a worthwhile
endeavor and time well spent writing this.

And so goes our life. I am done with the
book because I have no more to say that is
not repeating what I have already told
you. Life sucks and then you die. It is the
battle in between birth and death that
makes you the person that you are. It's
the trying to keep a loved one or yourself
from dying. It is getting up when life
keeps beating you down. Life is rarely
easy. Cancer is never easy. Loving
someone is always hard. But if you love
each other enough, you can beat anything

in your path. Cancer included.

If you are a husband reading this, love
your wife. If she has cancer or anything
else wrong with her, now is not the time
to put your marriage on hold while you
get through it. Now is the time to make
your marriage work for you like it always
has or maybe better than it ever has. Now
is the time to find her beautiful and sexy.
Now is the time to dance in the kitchen as
you make her dinner. Now is the time to
talk to her and listen to her more than you
ever have before.

If you are a wife reading this, realize how
much your husband loves you and what
he is going through inside just to be by
your side every day. As a man, our
greatest instinct is to protect and provide.
In this situation, we can't really do either
much of the time. And it eats at us inside.
A husbands goal is to keep on loving, to
keep on trying, to keep on fighting by
your side, we will do anything and go
through anything. Mike out.

ABOUT THE AUTHOR

Mike is a loving and dedicated husband to his wife Jennifer of 14 years and father to his furry children. When not taking care of Jen or hanging out in hospitals, he works as a scientist in pre-clinical research. He has also been a rugby player for twenty years which definitely gets the stress out.

www.ingramcontent.com/pod-product-compliance
Lightning Source LLC
Chambersburg PA
CBHW051449170526
45166CB00001B/172